Growing Up Pregnant

Growing Up Pregnant

A Young Woman's
Journey to Motherhood

Deirdre Curley

*This book is dedicated to my uncle Iain Campbell
and every young mother out there who has a dream*

Growing Up Pregnant: A Young Woman's Journey to Motherhood

First published in Great Britain in 2017 by Pinter & Martin

Copyright © Deirdre Curley 2017

ISBN 978-1-78066-435-4

Also available as ebook

Editor: Emma Grundy-Haigh
Additional editor: Anna Byrom
Proofreader: Sarah Dronfield

Waterfalls on page 6 © Gary Curley 2017, reproduced by kind permission

A CIP catalogue record for this book is available from the British Library.

Set in Dante

Printed in the UK by Martins the Printers Ltd.

This book has been printed on paper that is sourced and harvested from sustainable forests and is FSC accredited.

Pinter & Martin Ltd
6 Effra Parade
London SW2 1PS

www.pinterandmartin.com

You have to take risks. We will only understand
the miracle of life when we allow the unexpected to happen.

Paulo Coelho

Waterfalls

Waterfalls are everywhere –
We never know what they mean,
Until you jump into the blue,
And float into the stream.
Too scared to jump, because it's a long way down and in between.
I know what you're waiting for –
You've never been here before.

You left your parachute on the other side of town.
You know it's time to face the fear
And shake this solid ground.
Too scared to jump because it's a long way down and in between.
I know what you're waiting for –
You've never been here before.

Hold your breath and shut your eyes.
This is the change coming.
No time to back out of it now –
This is your time coming.
Never look back, never look back, never look back,
This is your waterfall.

The heart knows where to go but first you have to let go
Of all the things that keep you stuck in this old melting snow.
Still scared to jump because it's a long way down and in between.
Don't know what you're waiting for –
Well, you've been here before.

Unchartered waters and horizons never seen.
Open your eyes and walk the roads you've never been:
Don't be scared to jump because it's a long way down and in between.
Because if you do what you've always done,
You'll always have what you always had.

Hold your breath and shut your eyes.
This is the change coming.
No time to back out of it now –
This is your time coming.
Never look back, never look back, never look back,
This is your waterfall.

Gary Curley

PART 1

From Party Time Through the First Trimester

She's Leaving Home

When I was growing up on the Isle of Skye, there was a story going around that in the 1970s a girl packed her bag, took off on her bicycle and cycled all the way from Skye to Paris. She returned five years later, full of tales of love, friendship and adventure. Being a bit of a dreamer myself, this story got under my skin, inspiring me to believe that I too could go it alone, and that's exactly what I did at the tender age of sixteen.

But I had a different agenda. I was passionate about pursuing an acting career, and my local school at that time did not have Drama on the curriculum. This was massively frustrating to me, because the only access I had to the stage as a young girl was taking part in the local annual pantomime, which I loved, but it wasn't enough when I knew there was a whole world out there waiting for me to burst onto stage. It took an awful lot to persuade my mum and dad that the wisest move was to let me go, that I could only accomplish my dream if I studied acting at college in Glasgow instead of going into my final year at school. From my mother's point of view, the most important aspect was to find me safe accommodation with people known to her, and so began the task to find a flat with a connection that she could relate to, and so have peace of mind. That duly happened, and after several phone conversations we found a room where she could envisage I would settle in.

On the day that I left home, I woke up to the sun blinding me through a gap in the curtains. My head was thumping from the night before. I had been surreptitiously given a cocktail by my brother, to celebrate this new chapter in my life. With my head spinning, I realised that the malt whiskies had ended up being vomited onto the carpet of my sister's bedroom where I had crashed out. This was definitely not the leaving gift I had planned for her!

I heard my name being called from downstairs and realised I was late for my lift to my new life in Glasgow. The car had been packed the night before, with as much bedding and utensils as we could fit. Over an hour later, my head was still thumping. After goodbye hugs from all the family, I stumbled like a newborn calf towards the car and sidled into the passenger seat beside my mother, who was giving me the evils and impatient to make a start to the journey. I rolled down the window and hung my head out like a dog, hoping for even a spit of rain to moisten my dehydrated mouth. My new life wasn't getting off to the best of starts and to add insult to injury, I had to get my mum to stop in several lay-bys during the five-hour car journey. I received no sympathy from my frustrated mother, who was clearly wondering if this was a good idea after all.

It was approaching nightfall when we arrived at my new flat in Glasgow, a few hours later than planned. I looked out of the car window at bustling streets, neon lights, busy traffic and rows of tenement flats. It was a massive contrast to the tranquillity of Skye and the lonely house on the hill where I grew up. There, my neighbours were sheep and buzzards and midgies. I was going to have human neighbours for the first time in my life and this got my adrenalin pumping big time! My mum and I unloaded the car and we made my bedroom as homey as possible, taking note of what essentials were still missing, to be bought the next day.

I tried to settle for a much-needed sleep but the unfamiliar noises emanating from the surrounding flats kept me awake. I was on overdrive. I could hardly contain my excitement and nerves. I could hear people chattering, footsteps walking across floorboards, the sound of clanking pots and pans as people made their dinner. I got up and looked out my bedroom window. Across the street in the flat opposite I could see a young man hanging out his window puffing on a cigarette. I glanced at some of the other windows and could see that a party was in full swing. This was to become my life! Down the street I noticed that the bus shelter had been vandalised. Some people were mucking about there, quite aggressively, and I tried my best to listen in. Although I had fought hard to convince my parents that I was ready to go it alone, I had a wobble in my stomach and I could tell that nerves were setting in. I was here to start a new life and follow my dream of acting but even the performer in me started to get stage fright as the reality began to set in. I was here in the city, alone.

When Mum arrived the next morning to take me shopping, I didn't show her any of my concern. That would have been too risky. I might have been taken straight back up the road, and then what? A year of stalemate and boredom, not making any progress? Having to waste a precious year of my young and exciting new life? No way was that going to happen! We spent our last day together, finishing with a great meal in one of the best restaurants in the West End of the city. My mum and I still laugh at the significance of this meal, as it really did feel like the last supper. Her parting gift to me was a student cookbook. I didn't get around to opening it once during my spell as a student. My diet consisted instead of Super Noodles, microwavable meals, alcohol and anything in the 'deals' lane at Iceland. This was a million miles away from the wholesome meals cooked for us at home.

Say Hello to Your New Life

I soon realised after spending some time living alone that I hadn't fully thought things through. I was having to become responsible pretty much for the first time in my life. I was practically like a baby. I had to learn how to feed myself, how to do my own laundry, clothe myself and get to class on time without anyone yelling at me and telling me when to get up. It wasn't easy, but it had its benefits. I was having the time of my life. I could play my music as loud as I wanted, I was meeting lots of new people who I thought would be life-long friends and I could stay out all night without getting into trouble. From this point on I was in charge of my life and I felt completely free for the first time ever.

I had only spent a few days in Glasgow before moving there. One of those days was for the acting audition for the course I had been accepted onto. Despite my initial apprehension on the first night it didn't actually take long for me to settle into the Glasgow way of life. Thankfully I met Sadie and Pixie, two girls from acting school who I instantly bonded with. We quickly became friends, as we were all fun-loving free spirits. The girls also knew Glasgow like the back of their hand, having grown up there, so I had two amazing guides to show me what life in the city was really like.

Pixie and Sadie were both eighteen so I was the baby of the group. They took me under their wing and the first thing on their list was to get me a fake ID so that I too could get into the pubs and clubs that they frequented. My new name (according to my fake ID) was Debbie Ferguson. Debbie, I decided, studied Economics at Glasgow University and was nineteen years old. Being an actress, I enjoyed the challenge of becoming Debbie Ferguson, convincing bouncers at various pubs and clubs that I was old enough to get in. Debbie was great for me. She gave me access to unlimited alcohol, gambling and dancing. Debbie learned quickly how to work the bar for free drinks. She knew that the shorter the skirt the less likely you would be to be asked for ID on the way into a club. I inhabited a twilight world of fun and laughter, making new friends along the way and eating toasties in the after-hours casinos for the very reason that they were the cheapest in town. I was in my element and I became hooked on Glasgow's amazing music and arts scene. I was having the time of my life, and I hoped that life would go on like this for ever.

After some time, I realised that the college course I was on wasn't quite meeting my expectations and I spent many days dreaming of what would be next. I had a lot of restlessness within me and a burning desire to get the most out of life. I wanted everything that life could offer and no stone was going to be left unturned. I spent hours looking for courses that matched my aspirations and my desire to push myself out of my comfort zone. Inspired by a book that I had read called *Acting Teachers of America*, I applied to study on a six-week intensive course in New York City at the Ward Acting Studio. There, Wendy Ward taught the Meisner technique, which is a form of method acting. Wendy had twenty-five years' experience working with Hollywood actors and actresses and the dreamer in me knew that I needed to aim high in order to have any hope of achieving anything in such a competitive industry. I carried on with my college acting course every day, hoping that I would wake up to a letter in the post telling me that I had been accepted to the summer course in New York. To be honest, I suspected that I had maybe aimed a little bit too high with this application but the fantasy kept me going through the long hard days of studying on a course that I was beginning to lose interest in.

Before I knew it I was halfway through the last term at college and one of the top 'A' students in the class. Although I was near top of the class, I wasn't taking my studies seriously and my poor attendance actually jeopardised my chances of being accepted into second year (you can thank Debbie for that). When I think back, I realise that I was probably a bit overstimulated with all the new experiences I was having. Although I thought I was responsible, I was still learning to look after myself and get to know who I really was. On the days I wasn't hung-over and actually made it to class, I would immerse myself in learning as much as I could but it wasn't enough to keep my interest in the course alive. I was having too much fun burning the candle at both ends and dreaming about the idea of going to New York.

When news finally came, it was a morning like any other. I made my way through my embarrassingly messy flat to make myself my usual breakfast of coffee and a Pop Tart, and saw something on the floor that looked out of place. It was a large envelope with a strange-looking stamp on it. My initial thought was that it had been posted through my door by accident but on closer inspection I realised it was addressed to me. I carried the envelope into the kitchen and sat down on the old tatty seat next to the window that overlooked the famous Byres Road. I realised that this was my response from the acting studio in New York. My heart beat faster and I could feel the butterflies in my stomach surge as I closed my eyes and fantasised about the prospect of beginning a new adventure in New York. With trepidation, I slowly opened the letter. What would be next for me?

New York, New York

To be an interesting actor – hell, to be an interesting human being – you must be authentic and for you to be authentic you must embrace who you really are, warts and all. Do you have any idea how liberating it is to not care what people think about you? Well, that's what we're here to do.

Sanford Meisner

The envelope, it turned out, contained my acceptance letter to the acting course. After months of dreaming about opening this letter, it was finally here. I was officially going to New York for a six-week course in the summer break! It was at this precise moment that I realised I was also going to have to find a way to pay for it. Not exactly great planning on my part! Although I was striving for independence, the only way I could realistically afford to take the course was to ask the Bank of Mum and Dad to help me out. This new adventure was going to be expensive and still being slightly irresponsible, I hadn't really thought about how I was going to actually pay for it all. Luckily my mum and dad agreed to give me half of what I needed as long as I would commit to somehow paying for the rest. I was over the moon that my parents were going to help me but the trip was only three months away and I was flat broke.

At that time, I was working weekends in a fashionable clothes shop in the city centre as a retail assistant. I was earning the minimum wage and although I was living the life of a poor student in terms of my diet, my new lifestyle was getting a bit out of control. I was going to have to curb my partying for a while and save pretty much every spare penny I earned in the months leading up to going away. This was a bitter pill to swallow as I didn't want to stop enjoying myself but it was a necessary evil and I knew it would be worth it.

Eventually the big day came. I couldn't believe I was actually going to spend the summer in New York City. I boarded the flight alongside my mother and my best friend, Sadie, who kindly wanted to accompany me to help me settle in during the first week. I felt like a tiny little fish heading off to a great big pond. I was also feeling the same sense of trepidation that I had on my first night in Glasgow, but like before, I didn't let the fear get to me. I decided that I was going to embrace it and enjoy every minute of this amazing opportunity.

I had never been in a more challenging environment than the one I found myself in during this course. I had to be more disciplined than I'd ever been in my life and for someone who at seventeen clearly lacked discipline it was exhausting but incredibly rewarding at the same time. The classes were set up in such a way that everyone depended on the professionalism and commitment of their peers to learn lines, commit to performances and truly give it their all. It was a lot of pressure but I was fully immersed in acting and I was loving it. I felt like I had crossed over into the professional acting world. It required twenty-four-hour involvement. I was learning scripts in Central Park at lunchtime, visiting plays in the evening, rehearsing break-ups with fellow acting students in bars across the city, learning lines on the morning commute and it all had to come from the heart. I had to commit to the method, get out of my own head and become fully present. The course was eye-opening and taught me a lot about trust and respect. It was an awakening – everything just felt like it made sense.

Being seventeen, I was also keen to experience what the New York nightlife had to offer. As the drinking age in New York is twenty-one, I had to take on a new persona yet again. Debbie Ferguson, the name on my UK fake ID, was only nineteen. Again I was helped out by a classmate who got me an old student card and had my picture added to it. My new alter ego was Diane Rutherford, five years my senior, an acting student at the New York Film School and she, like Debbie Ferguson, was a great girl. As Diane, I was able to get my first tattoo, attend music festivals, roof top parties, amazing bars and nightclubs, basically everywhere you don't want your seventeen-year-old going in New York. I was excited to be an actress, I loved New York City and I truly felt that I had found my calling.

As I made my way home to Harlem each night from the acting studio, I felt like I was walking onto the set of a music video or a movie. Kids were bursting pipes all over the streets, men were coming up to ask me if I wanted to buy sunglasses, yellow taxis were flying by, there were hot dog stands on each corner. Although I was brought up a country bumpkin whose past excitement came from picking whelks off the shore for pocket money, I had completely fallen in love with this city. There was something in the air in New York. To this day I still can't sum up how the city made me feel, but it was unlike anything I've ever felt.

At the studio I was surrounded by a group of committed students from all around the world who were also hoping to be in that top one per cent of actors who actually make it. Everyone studied really hard throughout the day and most had to work really hard through the night in order to pay for their tuition. Some of my colleagues even worked in strip clubs to have enough money to cling onto their dreams of becoming actors. Being quite young at the time, I was a little shocked to hear this, as I could tell that some of the girls didn't want to dance for sleazy men to earn money, but they were determined individuals who were willing to swallow their pride in order to pay for their training. It was a revelation.

Towards the end of my stay in New York, my mother phoned to say my acting tutor in Glasgow had contacted her. They wanted me back for second year on the promise that I made a fresh start and committed to better attendance. But by this time my heart was in New York. I felt at home there. I battled with my mum on the phone to try and convince her that I should stay but she wasn't convinced. The conversation went something like:

"Mum, please I love it out here. Wendy says I can stay and study with her."

"We think you're better off coming home and finishing your course in Scotland, then you can go back out."

"I'll get a part-time job which will help pay my fees and rent."

"Well, you aren't doing a great job at managing your finances out there at the moment. How can you spend $80 in one weekend at seventeen?"

"Oh, I am actually twenty-two over here."

"You're coming home."

She was concerned for my well-being as any mother would be and I had pretty much run out of money and my mum wasn't going to bail me out this time as she knew I'd been up to no good. I was left with no choice but to return to Glasgow. I had ventured out into the wilderness and found myself in New York, but now I was going home and I was a little bit heartbroken.

Having spent now weeks developing the Meisner technique,

I was more underwhelmed with my college course than ever. I felt like I was just going through the motions. I missed New York and the intensity of the life-changing experience I had just had. However, I finally got myself together and was cast in two short films. In the first, I played an addict; this was closely followed by my next role where I was cast as a stalker. It would seem the casting agents got a sense that I was unhappy and thought I was perfect for these roles. I auditioned for one of Scotland's best acting schools later that year, and I chose *This Be the Verse* by Philip Larkin as my monologue (*'They fuck you up, your mum and dad.'*). Perhaps that sums up how frustrated I was with my situation.

Love Makes You Crazy

You can't plan who you are going to fall in love with, or when. At eighteen, I didn't really know much about what real love was. I had been in a couple of relationships but they never seemed to last long. After each inevitable break-up, I would always feel sorry for myself and I began to think that I was just unlucky in love. I was a pretty hopeless romantic to be fair and I'd do self-engrossed things like write songs for my lost loves in my diary and sadistically play Damien Rice songs to myself as I cried my eyes out. At this point in my life, I had given up on the idea of truly falling in love. I read all the time that you needed to love yourself before you could fully love anyone else, so at this rate, I thought it was going to take some years before I would be ready to let anybody in. Or so I thought.

Despite missing New York, I started to really appreciate how great Glasgow was as a city again. It truly was an outstanding place. One of the things that really hooked me was the legendary music scene there. At eighteen, the scene had four important meanings for me: *parties, alcohol, good music and boys*. This was the best cocktail for any night out and I loved a good strong mojito. In the blur of one of those nights, a guy really caught my eye and like any great cocktail, he could mix well. He was the DJ at one of the clubs I used to go to.

The whole room revolved around him. I was addicted before he even knew who I was. I went to the club often and I hoped that one night I would catch his eye, but I think I went about it in the wrong way by dancing on the tables and drunkenly asking him to play my favourite songs. I was young and wild and he seemed to have it together so it was going to take some work, but I had time on my side.

"I want to marry him," I whispered to my friend Sadie one night beneath the loud music, pointing to him in the DJ box.

"Who doesn't, look at him, he even has a dog!" she replied.

"I think he might also have a girlfriend. That's the problem."

"If he didn't have a girlfriend there would be something wrong. Let it go. For now just keep dancing like that – it's bound to at least get someone's attention."

As the months went by, I got to know him a little and it seemed like my luck might be about to change when I learned that he had actually split up from his girlfriend. I began to take every opportunity to be in his company. From hanging posters around town for his club nights to being down at the front at all his gigs and inviting him along to all my nights out. To say that I was keen would be an understatement.

He ticked all the boxes on my wish list:

- Singer in a band
- DJ
- Man not boy
- Whisky drinker
- Owned a car
- Incredibly handsome
- Funny
- Can stay up longer than me
- Not ashamed to eat Chinese at 3am (and perhaps the leftovers the following day)

Eventually it looked like I might be in with a shot when

he tentatively agreed to go out on a date with me. To be fair, I think he either gave in out of sympathy or perhaps he was worried that I might follow him around for the rest of his life if he didn't give me a chance. On our first date, we went to the cinema where we watched *Juno* (the irony of this was not lost on us later) and shared an ice cream. To me, this was progress. We shared the same spoon and everything! Over the coming months we fell more and more for each other. It was outside our control: there seemed to be an energy that drew us both together, and everyone in the room could feel it. We took things slowly in the beginning and neither of us was really looking for a commitment, but the connection we had was undeniable.

As our time together grew from weekends to almost every day of the week, we both began to become intrigued as to what a future together might look like. One day we visited a dogs' home and took a couple of the dogs out for a walk. We both loved dogs, as we both had grown up around them, and I often think we were doing this just to test out what it might feel like to have something that was ours to look after together. That said, we certainly didn't mention the word *baby*. We just seemed to enjoy the fifteen-minute commitment of walking a dog together, feeling good about it and knowing that we could pop it safely back into its kennel when we were ready to go.

Thinking back to the relationships I had been in before I instinctively knew that this one was different. I was young but this wasn't young love. This *was* love. The man I thought was just good at spinning tunes, performing in a band and being great at being handsome was also a smart, kind, loving, hilarious, adventurous soul, searching, as I was, for a soulmate.

I was ready to upgrade my Facebook status to 'in a relationship' – that's proper confirmation, right? I decided to spend my savings on a surprise trip to Europe. I booked Oslo, a few hours' plane journey from Glasgow with return prices for less than I spend on a night out. I thought it would be a good cheap place to have some romantic fun. An unusual destination, which I thought might appeal to my boyfriend. A few drinks later, we landed in Oslo and got into a taxi where the confused driver began to quiz us.

"Why are you here?" he asked, smiling at us.

"I just wanted to surprise my boyfriend," I said innocently.

"No one your age comes here."

"Why?" I asked, confused, as we sat in the back of the taxi.

"This place is one of the most expensive cities in Europe."

Shit.

"Where would you like me to take you?" he asked.

"I haven't actually booked any accommodation – just anywhere cheap," I replied, scanning my Gary's worried look.

"That's the problem, there is nowhere cheap in Oslo," the taxi driver said.

Despite the look of worry on Gary's face, we both began to see the funny side of our predicament and instead of panicking we started to laugh uncontrollably. We were dropped off in a beautiful square and began our search for accommodation. Everywhere cost as much for one night as I had saved up for the entire trip. Yes, I had actually saved up for something – at least that was fairly responsible.

"Wait here," Gary said. "I've got an idea!"

I waited patiently outside what looked like Oslo's version of *Fawlty Towers*. Suddenly I heard someone shouting something from up above. It was Gary and he was signalling me that he was in room 206. I entered the hotel and sneaked into one of the lifts. When I arrived at room 206 I chapped on the door and Gary opened it to reveal a tiny single bed overlooking the square. We started to laugh again, thinking that this was perhaps the worst room in the whole of Oslo.

When Gary had enquired at reception, he realised that we could only afford a single room, so I spent the remaining three days of the trip sneaking in and out of room 206. It was hilarious really and all down to my bad planning. I really had no idea Oslo was the most expensive city in Europe.

A lot of our days back home were spent driving around. He was like a tour guide and patiently showed me around the city he grew up in. He was a proper city kid and I was an islander attempting to be a city kid. Every day was different and always had a great soundtrack. The day we pulled up to go for a walk in the woods was perhaps one of the most profound of them all. We walked through a dark forest trail, until we could hear the sound of a waterfall in the distance. As we approached, we heard laughter in the air. Reaching the top of the hill we looked down on a beautiful waterfall with a glorious pool of water beneath. It was an unusually sunny day by Scottish standards and we watched as people jumped off the top of the waterfall to swim in the pool below.

"Why don't we join them?" he said clasping my hand.

"Are you kidding me?" I replied.

"I think we should jump in. It looks like fun."

"But we didn't bring proper swimming stuff."

"Who cares, neither did half of the people in there. Let's just go for it, it looks safe and the worst that could happen is we get a little wet. It's so warm that we'll dry off quickly. Let's get over our fear."

We stared for a few minutes and I began to question myself. Should I jump in? Would it be really cool if I do this? Was he seeing this as a sign, that if we jump in together we will last? In the end we chickened out. We walked away and I spent the rest of the day wishing we had jumped, wishing I could have been brave, wishing that I had embraced the moment more.

That summer I had already arranged to go back to Skye to earn money at the local hotel, so Gary and I ended up spending some time apart. During that phase, I tried to figure out what the universe might have in store for me next. Gary also took some time out to focus on his music and visit his parents who lived abroad. My mother knew it was beginning to get serious when a monstrous phone bill came in. I had inadvertently spent a lot of money on phone calls to Abu Dhabi where Gary was staying. So much for my savings. Most of it went on paying for the phone bill! Our time apart that summer only served to make us feel closer than ever. It's an old cliché but absence did make our hearts grow even fonder and so one day I made an impromptu decision to grab a lift to Gary's parents house in Glasgow that he was living in while they were abroad. I was missing him too much. I forgot to ask if I could move in with him, I just did.

It wasn't unlike us to throw caution to the wind. Some days we would go for a drink in Glasgow and end up four hours south in random places like Blackpool. We just went with the flow and seemed to always bring out the spontaneity in each other. We were quite a whimsical pair and enjoyed pointing out the various signs we were seeing that we thought confirmed we were meant to be with each other. The night we discovered matching moles on identical parts of our left arm in a motel in Blackpool was a particular highlight, and we agreed that this was further evidence of our destiny to be together. We didn't need rings on our fingers to confirm our love, we had matching moles! We celebrated this discovery by running barefoot across a windy Blackpool beach in the pitch dark. Later we found ourselves gatecrashing a line dancers' trip, and ended up sipping drinks into the early hours with men and women in their eighties. I spent the next few days wondering if we had known each other in a past life and somehow had these moles so that we would know how to find each other in this life. I think it's true what they say: love really does make you crazy!

Weeks turned into months and I knew things were moving to the next level when I got the invitation of a lifetime. I was to visit his parents in Abu Dhabi where they worked. I felt like I had won the golden ticket! There I was boarding a flight to the desert sands and sun, leaving my welly boots and waitressing job behind for a blissful two weeks of exploring the desert, soaking up a new culture and getting to know his family. I must admit, I really felt like I was going places! We had a lot of fun on that holiday, maybe too much!

Mystic Meg

I was settling into my new life as a full-time girlfriend but still spent many hours of my days searching for answers. What was my calling? What did the universe have in store for me next? Was it acting, my first love and the thing that made me feel most alive and in the moment? Was it writing? Gary was kind and said that I had a creative soul that was trying to emerge after he stumbled upon the songs and poems I used to write in my diary. Was it my dream to open a bar? Maybe not a great idea for someone who clearly enjoyed the good life as much as I did. Was it to book a round-the-world ticket and go away to find myself? I had so many options, the world was my oyster. I was in love and I was ready to have it all. During a moment of existential panic, I took the bus to a local psychic. I wanted more signs. Some guidance. I needed some kind of insight into my future because although I seemed sure of myself to the outside world, I really didn't know who I was yet. I was hoping that the psychic could give me clarification on what lay ahead – kind of ridiculous I know!

The psychic was located in an old rundown community centre in the heart of one of Glasgow's least glamorous areas. As I made my journey over on that miserable Scottish day, I closed my eyes and put myself back on the sandy beach I lay on just two weeks before, hoping it would warm me, remind me of the peace I felt and the hope I had that my life was going to be one of real meaning. Aside from all the other nonsense I was told by Mystic Meg that day, she said something that sounded completely ridiculous. Someone close to me was pregnant. I laughed out loud as I went through my friends and sisters one by one trying to weigh up who it could be. There was no way any of them could be pregnant. I even entertained the thought for a second that it could have been Mystic Meg herself that was pregnant – she was close to me after all – right across the table, in fact! I left the psychic centre and decided to text my friends for a laugh, saying that the psychic told me that one of them may be pregnant. An outpouring of worried replies followed and some of them actually took a pregnancy test! I felt a little bit bad for worrying my friends, but it was the one thing that the psychic said that had a small chance of being true so I felt like it was my duty. Some of the replies read:

I have just taken the test, I am all clear. Shame I've caught an STD though. That sucks. Only kidding.

I'm still a virgin. LOL.

My ex-boyfriend is going to be so mad when he finds out I am carrying his baby. Joke, but you owe me a drink this weekend, what a thing to put me through!

The weeks passed, and the penny began to drop. My period was now two days late and it was two weeks since Mystic Meg cast her spell upon me. I remember it like it was yesterday. It was a freezing December day and I woke up next to my Gary in a cold panic, rushing out of bed to the bathroom to look for a sign of my late period. Still nothing. Imagine if it was me! We had not long been visiting his parents in a different time zone abroad. Had I not taken my pill on time? Had I accidentally missed the twelve-hour window or even missed a pill completely? How could I be so irresponsible? You are pretty cruel to yourself when you are terrified. So please note, it's natural.

I continued sinking into a state of deep anxiety. After confirming on Google that perhaps my period hadn't arrived due to 'stress' I eventually plucked up the courage to wander to the local chemist. Thankfully, because I was an 'outsider' in Erskine where Gary lived nobody really knew me in the area yet, so I was confident I wouldn't bump into someone I knew and have to lie about why I was there. I pulled my beanie hat as far down my face as possible and entered the shop. I knew that I shouldn't have felt embarrassed but I was. Embarrassed and terrified. It was excruciating. Like the first time I had to enter a chemist for Tampax at sixteen. I now know that I shouldn't have been so hard on myself but I was young and scared. As I picked up the pregnancy test from the counter and placed it down on the till, I received an unforgettable look from the nerd behind the counter and hung my head in shame. I left the shop and began the long walk home. *Not the walk of shame I was used to.* During my walk home to my boyfriend's house with the pregnancy test safely hidden in my handbag, I reflected over the past few weeks, trying to work out if there were any signs of pregnancy. Have I felt more tired than usual? Were my boobs getting bigger? I always wanted bigger boobs but in this moment I really hoped that they hadn't changed. My emotions were all over the place. I was going between episodes of laughter, fear and dread. It felt like I was taking a long walk off a short plank into the unknown.

I began to argue with myself:

What if I am pregnant?

I'm going to have to google ways to make this stop.

Calm down, you haven't even taken the test.

I remember there's a part in Juno *where she pretends she is going to kill herself.*

It's only a baby, calm down.

A baby? *Only* a baby? *What the hell am I going to do with a* baby? *I'm still learning to look after myself!*

I really want a cuddle from my mum right now.

She's probably going to give you hell for this.

How will I tell him if I am?

He is going to freak out! He is going to leave you!

I'm going to have to get an abortion!

What am I going to do?

You are not *pregnant, stop worrying.*

I arrived back at my Gary's house and quickly checked inside the fridge for some wine to calm my nerves. Then I thought to myself, *Stop. You can't drink that if you're pregnant!* It was crazy and it was all starting to feel very real in that moment. It's amazing how effectively panic can come crashing down into the present moment! My whole future was hanging in the balance now. Was this really what the universe had in store for me next? Surely not. I opened the door into the downstairs bathroom and giggled nervously to myself. Why was I panicking so much? For a moment I felt a fleeting sense of relief as I thought to myself that I might actually *not* be pregnant! Wouldn't that be hilarious! I'd need to come up with a plan to ditch the test in a bin far away so that I don't scare him off. Yes, everything *might* be OK!

I unwrapped the box and looked at the test like it was the most unwanted Christmas gift in the pile. I followed the instructions, lowered the test into the toilet and began to pee all over my hand. Taking a pregnancy test certainly isn't the most glamorous of activities and I couldn't stop shaking. I was so scared! The next two minutes were possibly the longest in my life, as I stared at the test in stunned silence waiting for the result.

And there it was. Staring right back at me. That little pink line! I *was* pregnant! There are three common reactions to that tiny innocent pink line on a pregnancy test.

"We did it, I'm pregnant!"

"Well, I guess there's no such thing as 'the right time' is there?" and

"Oh shit, what the hell do I do now!?"

I will leave it up to you, dear reader, to decide what my reaction was.

I was about to turn nineteen and I'd only been dating the love of my life for about nine months. How ironic was it that it would take the same amount of time to become parents. I joked to myself that it wasn't a pregnancy test I actually needed now, it was Harry Potter's wand – because at this point, the only thing that could change the reality of the result was real magic!

Living Life in Reverse

I had always wanted to be older than my age. Growing up, some of my life goals were:

- When I turn sixteen, I can get my belly button pierced.
- When I turn eighteen, I can buy alcohol.
- When I turn twenty-one, I can gamble in Vegas.

I always felt that growing up was such a long process. I always looked forward to the next milestone. I was always searching for something more and hoping that time would pass quickly so that I could be older, more responsible, more in control. Even at the age of five, I wanted to be more grown up. I can remember donning a tiny uniform and making my way down to the local hotel for my pretend reception job, much to the amusement of everyone who witnessed it. I spent many school nights praying that I would wake up and it would magically be my last day so that I could leave and start my real life. And, as you know, I later enjoyed pretending to be older than my years so that I could gain entry into nightclubs, tattoo parlours and pubs. Up until now, I had experienced momentary flashes of what it felt like to be present and in the moment but for the most part I was always focusing on what was next. But now, for the first time in my whole life, I found myself truly living in the present moment and unable to picture what the future might look like.

I CAN'T BELIEVE IT! I AM ACTUALLY PREGNANT!

I found myself now wishing the clocks would stop – maybe even turn back. I was so confused as I tried to look inward for answers perhaps for the first time in my eighteen years. I had always looked outside of myself for signs and answers. I was mortified about the position I had got myself and my boyfriend into. I felt responsible for becoming pregnant, as I was on the pill. Gary also knew I was on the pill. I couldn't fathom how this had happened. I was dreading the moment he was to return home from his DJ gig and I would have to break the news to him. It wasn't just the surprise and shock of the result that was worrying me. I had witnessed the way society judges young women who get pregnant and have children at a younger age. Back in my mum's day, nineteen was actually a pretty normal age to get pregnant, but today the societal ideas of a 'normal' age to begin a family seem to have shifted from starting when you are young to it being more normal to have a baby later in life. I did some more googling and found out that most people seemed to think your mid-thirties was the 'best' time to have children, once you had a career, a home, a husband, etc. *I don't even have a driver's licence. What am I going to do with a baby?*

As I evaluated my situation, I came to the conclusion that going through with this pregnancy was probably the wrong thing to do. It wasn't the right time. I had so little to offer a new life, I decided. The closest thing I had to a career was a part-time job as a waitress at the local pizza restaurant that I had recently picked up. I was living at Gary's parents house and although we loved each other, we'd never even talked about getting married never mind having children. We wouldn't be doing things in the 'correct' order if we had this baby – another societal pressure. It was so far from what I thought we both wanted. Also, I actually *had* to break the news to Gary. I was

going to have to tell him, *"Surprise!* You're going to be a father!"
I had no choice. I wasn't going to end up on *Jeremy Kyle*. I began
to feel very inadequate and insecure. I could barely throw a
meal together, how was I going to be able to look after another
person? *Yes*, I thought, *this is never going to work out. I'm just not
capable of becoming a parent.*

Gary and I were still very much in the honeymoon stage
of our relationship. It was full force. We spent most of our
time dreaming up cool adventures to go on, finding unusual
places to have sex or driving around in his car listening to The
Smiths and talking about our dreams of working full-time in
the creative industries one day. One of our most prominent and
shared dreams was to lead a fun, adventurous, bohemian life.
A 'John and Yoko' kind of life. With the outside possibility of
maybe having a few dogs in a couple of years to really show our
commitment to each other.

Suddenly I realised that the baby that was growing inside
me wasn't only about me. This result was *our* result. Gary was
the father. I began to wonder what he really thought of me
and whether he was truly happy with me. When he found
out, would he wish that we had never met? Would he regret
allowing me to move in with him? Would he wish that he had
never actually found me the day that I had planned a treasure
hunt across Glasgow that led him to a hotel room where I had
wrapped myself up in an Ann Summers box! Maybe he would
wish that I had never returned from New York, that he hadn't
driven 250 miles just to see me one night when I was in Skye
when he was missing me. I wondered if he really wanted more
time to be free, to go and figure it all out for himself, like I was
trying to do.

I wondered what I could say that would soften the blow.
I had literally just learned that you don't stick knives in your

toaster and that you don't stare into a microwave when it's heating up your dinner. I had just mastered at what point you fill your Pot Noodle up to with boiling water, so as not to ruin it. I had just come to terms with the fact that you need to pay for electricity, heating and council tax when you decide to leave home and your parents stop paying your way. I had just grasped that banks *want* you to take out credit cards so that you spend your life in crippling debt. I doubt very much that he had ever thought of me as the mother of his child. I was just a girl finding her way in this world, slowly, but surely.

When it came down to the crunch, despite all the feelings of inadequacy and panic, I realised that I did actually want to have his child. I wanted all of him. I wanted him to wrap me up in his arms and tell me that everything was going to be fine and that we would take it one day at a time and that no matter what happened, or what people said, we would get through it. I wanted him to laugh and say that it was just another sign, another reason why we were destined to be together. I wanted him to tell me that it wasn't my fault. I wanted him to tell me that one day, when it was all figured out, we could move to New York so that I could finish my acting training, because having children shouldn't get in the way of your dreams and we'd bring our child up the best way we could, with what we had. I wanted him to tell me to stop crying so much, to stop feeling sick with worry, to just stop and look him in the eyes and trust him that we were going to get through all of this together. I wanted him to say that nothing was going to change and that even though we weren't engaged yet, he would one day marry me because he did truly love me and he always would and that he would love and protect our family through any turbulence we came across in our life. I was hoping for him to say a lot in that moment!

But that's exactly what he did say.

It's OK Not to Be OK

Nothing quite prepares you for the moment when something that cost you 99 pence from a local chemist turns into something that will potentially cost you approximately £200,000 over the next twenty-one years. A new baby will cost you a lot. It's one of the biggest investments you will ever make, not just financially but physically and mentally as well. I can understand why some couples never seem to find the 'right time' to have a baby, because when you think it through logically it can seem like a very daunting and scary prospect. So, if you find yourself to be pregnant and it is in fact unplanned, you really need to give yourself permission to be human. It's a huge thing to process when you are not prepared, so it's OK not to be OK.

I began to write down my thoughts, all the pros and cons of going through with this and bringing a child into the world. On reflection, they seem a little shallow and selfish but again you need to give yourself permission to be a little bit irrational if you weren't expecting to be expecting. My thoughts went a little like this:

Positives
- I'll be a young mother
- It might motivate me to do more
- I'll not have a period for nine months
- Our parents will love to be grandparents (hopefully)
- It'll be an adventure

- We will be showing commitment to each other
- My boobs might get bigger
- It will give me motivation to be a better actress

Negatives
- I can't party for nine months
- My acting career is over before it's even begun
- What if the baby doesn't like me?
- My body is never going to be the same again
- My vagina is ruined
- I'm going to have to get my tits out in public
- How will I afford nursery fees?
- I'll need to get a proper job
- I'm going to have stretch marks
- No one is going to want to be my friend

Everything was new to me, to us. We knew that we were in love, but were we really ready to become parents? I had never been attracted to babies, by which I mean I didn't get all weak at the knees at the sight of newborns like some of my friends did. I didn't understand why people babbled incomprehensibly to babies and sang to them two pitches higher than was necessary as if it was normal. I had only really held one baby in my life when I was around eight years old. A ten-day-old baby girl. She looked me straight in the eye and was sick all over my favourite jumper. Everyone in the room just went 'Awwww' like she was throwing up candyfloss. Between this notorious event and a recurring nightmare of dying during childbirth, pregnancy had never been at the forefront of my mind.

Being the inquisitive type I had observed mothers for years. First my own and then others in real life and in movies, like it was a role in life that I was never going to be ready for. A role for older, much wiser women. Mothers to me seemed to have a lot of responsibilities and I had always been fairly irresponsible. The mothers I knew were so busy and seemed to be in charge of everything in their households from the cooking, cleaning, school runs and washing-up, etc. The only part that I could look forward to would be when I could put on fancy dress to play the Tooth Fairy or Santa Claus. My mother was the absolute world to me when I was a child. How could I possibly do all this?

I started to wonder why I felt like I was doing something wrong by deciding to have my baby. Was this not what life was all about? Why was I worried that I was not ready to become a mother? I took some comfort in the fact that Gary's mother was only twenty-one when she had her first child, but being a mum at nineteen still seemed daunting. My head raced as I thought about all the people who were going to judge me, like some of my younger friends who were only months out of school. I also began to think about how many people I might hurt when I broke the news that I was having a baby. The pressure began to overwhelm me. For the first time in my life I felt like I was growing up too fast.

Each morning I woke up and tried to tune in to what was happening inside my body. I was concerned about the development of the baby and wondered if I was doing all the right things. Whether I was eating enough food or drinking enough fluids. As the weeks passed, I felt I had less energy than I used to. There were no other clear signs that I was pregnant though, as I wasn't experiencing any morning sickness yet. At certain points in the weeks after the pregnancy test, I actually wondered if I should take another one just to make sure that the first one was correct. I hid in my bedroom and called the doctor's surgery in Glasgow, readying myself to tell the first person outside of Gary that I was pregnant. It started to feel real during that phone call.

Gary and I spent Christmas and New Year at home with my family on Skye who had no idea what was going on yet. I remember obsessively looking up job sites and hoping that the New Year would bring me a better job as well as a healthy baby.

As I was usually known as the driving force behind instigating parties and staying up all night, I also had to make up some creative excuses so that no one would wonder why I was always heading to bed early. I was enjoying being able to relax and laze around in my pyjamas all day while my mum looked after me. She could tell that I wasn't my usual energetic self. Mothers always know when something is going on. I was enjoying spending time with her but I was also terrified that I'd start being sick and blow my cover! It was Gary and my first Christmas together as a couple and at some points I completely forgot that I was carrying a baby as I involved myself in various conversations with my parents about my future. I spoke of my ambition to get a good agent and try to get into a play at the Fringe Festival that year.

I'd almost convinced myself that this was going to happen but then I would remember that I'd probably be learning how to change nappies and not learning lines by the time the Fringe came to Edinburgh next year. Their encouragement to chase my dreams, whatever they had been at the time, was always something I admired about my parents. If I wanted to be an astronaut that would have been OK, but being a mother at nineteen, I wasn't sure if that would get the same support.

I spent a lot of that festive period being around another important man in my life, my uncle. He had experienced his fair share of challenging moments in life, the biggest one being his cancer diagnosis four years before. He was the one who had thrown the best parties when I was growing up, the one who would take time out of his day to really listen to me although I'm sure he had much better things to do.

He was now in the final year of his expected time and we spoke for hours over the holidays about the true meaning of life. During these long talks, I was acutely aware of the new life growing inside me. I felt a profound sense of sorrow knowing that his life was dwindling away. He was someone who had learned to give all the power to the present moment. He taught me that it's best to let go of the past and try to live fully in the now because it's all we really have. This poignant advice helped me find strength within myself in facing the reality of my pregnancy and the fact that I was going to become a mother.

The days started to fly by and January was now on my doorstep. It was time for my first doctor's appointment. I sat down in the doctor's office and told her my story. My emotions were high during the consultation and I began to weep as she wrote down the date of my last period and made her calculation. She told me that my baby was due on 18 August. The first thing I did was to calculate the months that my uncle might still be here for. It looked promising that he would get to meet my baby when it arrived into the world.

"I will make an appointment with your local midwife who will get you booked in for your first scan and your screening tests over the next few weeks. They will also schedule in your antenatal classes," the doctor said.

"Thank you," I replied.

"Are you pleased with your decision to have a baby?"

"Eh, yes, yes, I am."

"Great, does your partner know?"

"Yes, he does."

"Good, now please come back to see me if there is anything else you need."

The hardest decisions I had had to make before deciding to have a baby were things like whether I would wear boots or heels on a night out, whether I would have jam or peanut butter on my toast or if I should have cranberry or diet coke as a mixer with my vodka! Now I was faced with deeply confusing questions like whether or not I was able, capable or even brave enough to look after, love and protect this small life growing inside me. Gary and I had a feeling that, despite the initial panic and soul searching, everything would somehow be OK. Sometimes when you're not sure what to do, you have to trust your feelings. Neither Gary nor I were sure what to expect, but we were sure that we had enough love for each other to make it work.

Like Mother Like Daughter

I spent a lot of time thinking of my own mother in the first few months of pregnancy. Rarely focusing on the fear of telling her (that came later). Now that I was going to be a mother myself, I began to see and appreciate her from a whole new perspective. She had spent the past twenty-four years raising five children. Five children! That to me now seemed like an amazing feat. I was still freaking out over the idea of bringing one into the world.

My mum had been a pretty cool kid. An art student in Glasgow in the seventies she was also a bit of a party animal. She too loved the art and music scene in Glasgow. She would eventually meet and marry my dad. Another musician. Just like Gary. I clearly couldn't wait to be just like her.

I remember her reminiscing about her adolescent years, which were spent practically imprisoned in an all girls' boarding school in Aberdeenshire hundreds of miles away from her parents. She was sent away to boarding school when she was eleven years old against her wishes. She was happy in her own wee world at home on Skye and really didn't want to leave. Her world, like mine when I was a child, was full of serenity and beauty, surrounded by flowing rivers, moors and wild flowers. She felt defeated when it became clear that her voice wasn't going to count for anything. Her parents were in charge and they had decided that she was going to boarding school. She began to kick back against the move almost immediately. When the girls at the school were told to write their first letter home, my mother didn't mince her words about how unhappy she was. However, all the letters were vetted by the housemistress before being posted and she was told to rewrite the letters until it sounded like she was content there. As the years progressed, she and a small group of friends started to plot ways to add a little bit of excitement to the routine and discipline they were subjected to day in day out. Soon they were sneaking out to rock concerts late at night after lights out. They concocted an ingenious plan to sneak back in with the morning rolls delivery at around 6am. It was a bit of a gamble but as luck would have it, the driver turned out to be a good sport and went along with the plan. It seemed like the perfect plan until it wasn't about three escapes later when they were caught red-handed and she was sent back home to Skye, exactly where she wanted to be.

As a child growing up on Skye, I loved how beautifully raw life was. Most mornings I was thrown out to the elements, to spend time on the seashore picking whelks and fishing for crabs and mackerel off the pier before heading around the local village to sell my fish to anyone who felt sorry for me. There wasn't a day that went by that something miraculous didn't happen, like watching otters walk out of the sea up to our doorstep. Every day there was a miracle of nature; we were blessed to be part of it all. But as I got into my teens, I began to crave freedom. As much as I loved Skye, it was too quiet for me.

Over the early years, my mum was the glue that held us all together, she was just bloody lovely. Five children weren't enough for her; all our friends would be welcomed into our home with open arms. Our adventurous childhood took us to all the corners of Scotland. Treasure hunts in the Borders, dance routines in Dornoch, drama classes in Eden Court, papermaking in Helmsdale, you name it – we turned up! She was up for anything. As I compared the childhood that my parents gave us to the one that I could give this baby, I became more and more anxious. I didn't have a car to drive, a proper job with maternity cover or any experience looking after children; I didn't even have a ring on my finger. All the things most mothers have, or so you're led to believe.

Anxiety was a familiar feeling to me, having had many bouts of it growing up. One of those bouts was about deciding which book I was going to pick for my English exam three years previous. Although I wanted to be an actress, studying William Shakespeare, despite encouragement from my teachers, just wasn't my *thing*. So my mother took it upon herself to find the perfect book for me to study, one which I could relate to, and most importantly, one which I could pass my exam with. *Growing Up a Drunk Girl* by Koren Zailckas was the book she picked. Yes, I was only sixteen, but hey, I'd already raided the cocktail cabinet in the house for various camping trips and made efforts at my own home brew, so I had a rough idea of what the girl was writing about. I remember that on the last day of school I was so elated to finish school that my mother decided to enter into the sheer excitement that I was expressing by dumping all the school jotters in a heap and handing me a match in the garden. The bonfire of the century! It was one of the most liberating experiences of my life and I was so glad to be sharing it with her. She totally got me.

"When do you think you'll have children?" my mother asked during a heart-to-heart.

"Kids aren't really my thing, Mum. When I'm twenty-nine I think I might have changed my mind." This was my 'perfect age' to *consider* getting pregnant.

"Did you always want five kids, Mum? I mean, it's a bit crazy, isn't it?"

"When your big brother, John, was born, a light came on that had been stamped out by years of searching in the wrong places. My world changed the moment I held him in my arms for the first time. I looked at him and everything started to make sense. I felt a powerful sense of love unlike anything I had felt before. It was like he completed me. I had the same feeling of wonder when I had all my children. I'm so grateful to have known this love, this life force. I feel like it has sustained me and kept me going through all of life's ups and downs. We made many sacrifices in order to have such a big family, but it was one of the easiest decisions I have ever made once I knew what being a mother felt like."

What would I be sacrificing? My young body? My freedom? Spontaneous adventures? Sleep? Nights out with friends? My career? I'd crammed a whole lot of living into my eighteen years on this earth but now it was going to come to a complete standstill. What was I really giving up? It really didn't seem like much at all and there was one thing that I knew would stand me in good stead. My mother had blessed me with a kind heart. My 'potty mouth' on the other hand – well, you can thank my father for that.

Working 9–5

I thought it was a wise idea to start to present myself as someone who could be responsible before the news broke to the world that I was going to become a mum. My dreams of being picked up by a casting agent while in my current waitressing job seemed like a very unrealistic prospect now. I needed to get a real, grown-up job to prove to myself and others that I was moving forward with my life and that I could take care of myself. I was going to have to take care of a baby too, after all. Time was starting to work against me. Weeks were flying by quickly and I was painfully aware that in around four weeks my current flat stomach was going to be replaced by a visible bump. It was important to grab a position in some line of work before I had to announce that I was pregnant.

I went for a couple of interviews. One was for an admin position at one of the high street banks. The role involved spending eight hours a day on the phone chasing up people who hadn't paid their debts. I thought it would be nice to be on the other side of the phone call for once, so when I was offered the position I took the zero-hour contract. I didn't really have anything to lose at this point and I thought to myself that it would, at the very least, be better than a previous job I had: cold calling people to sell double-glazing. I was literally told to fuck off at least fifty times a day on that dire job. A typical morning went something like this:

"Would you like a drink to get you started dear?" the office waitress would shout across the office floor to me.

"What are the options?" I would reply.

"So we have vodka and coke for £2, glass of Buck's fizz for £1.50 or gin and tonic."

"How much is the gin and tonic?"

"Oh hen, I'm sorry but we've had to put the price of gin and tonic up to £1.55."

"That's fine, I will have one of each. That should see me through until lunch at 1pm."

I needed something to numb the excruciating horror of being verbally abused all day down the phone line. It really was the job from hell. I didn't think about it much at the time but I soon realised that chasing people up for unpaid debt would elicit the same kind of responses as cold calling them to sell windows! I didn't have any other options on the job front though and we needed the money. I was also hoping to impress my boss and work hard so that I could be issued a full-term contract.

I borrowed an appropriately ladylike dress from my sister's wardrobe and each day took the train journey from Erskine in to the city office. I loved the early-hour commute, the morning commuters all bustling in the streets grasping their cups of coffee and queuing up for their black pudding rolls. I felt as if I was becoming someone in the world. Or at least I tried to convince myself that I was. I imagined myself to be like a character from *Mad Men* rushing into the city office job with great purpose. One day, I arrived at the office and everyone was bundled into a small room. *Oh no*, I thought! *What now? Are we all going to be fired?*

"Half of you will be kept on after three weeks, so make sure you all do your best to reach the targets. If you don't, you will only be letting yourselves down and will probably be let go," my boss stated.

I gazed around the room and everyone looked miserable. I too felt a sense of dread. I really couldn't afford to lose this job. All of a sudden an overwhelming feeling of sickness came over me. I excused myself and ran to the washroom. I literally kicked the cubicle door open and vomited violently all over a closed toilet pan! It went everywhere! The explosive vomiting was followed by a few minutes of dry retching. When I was sure that there was no more, I got myself (and the toilet) cleaned up. I remember feeling glad that no one was sitting on that toilet when I kicked the door open, as they really would have been decorated head to toe with what I had had for breakfast that morning.

That was the first bout of morning sickness I had experienced. Talk about perfect timing.

Shit! I thought. *I've been in here for ten minutes. People are going to wonder what the hell I've been doing!* I attempted to fix my face before cautiously walking back into the office. I soon got over the initial shock of my experience in the toilet and began my work.

As the weeks went by, I made a great impression with my boss. I began being awarded employee of the week and smashing all my targets. It was such an incredible feeling. I felt like I was winning, like I was taking control and steering my life in the right direction. It also meant that I would hopefully have some guaranteed income in my bank, at least until the baby was born. All I had to do was keep doing what I was doing and make it through the next three weeks and a full-time contract would hopefully be offered.

Happy Birthday

It was coming up to midnight on the eve of my nineteenth birthday. I was now coming up to twelve weeks but still no one knew. I spent my birthday night out celebrating with a large group of friends and family at one of the clubs where Gary was DJing. In an effort to remain in character, I flushed the alcoholic drinks that had been bought for me down the toilet and bought myself soft drinks to give the illusion that I was actually drinking. I didn't want to make people suspicious by not drinking. I also fooled everyone by doing my usual dance routine on the tables to Amy Winehouse. "They tried to make me go to rehab," sang Amy. I felt like I was in rehab, as I was completely sober in a club for practically the first time in my life.

Twelve weeks in and I'd started to forget what being drunk felt like. I was putting on the best performance of my life *pretending* that I was thoroughly enjoying myself, *pretending* not to be terrified, while we all spun around dancing to The Bangles' 'Walk like an Egyptian' on the dance floor. Throughout the evening I was constantly reminded that I had a baby growing inside me as I needed to pee literally every twenty minutes and my boobs really hurt when people in the club accidentally bumped into me. That night I actually wanted nothing more than to be curled up in bed with a hot-water bottle instead of being in a club. Another first!

I kept looking over at Gary behind the decks from the dance

floor. It was here that we had first met around a year before. Occasionally I saw him lift his face up from behind the decks to try and catch my eye. A year ago, I was the one trying to catch his eye and now we were to be parents. We smiled at each other and it was like we didn't need to say anything. Our eyes did all the talking for us. Behind our smiles we were hiding some of the doubts and worries we both had. We were both putting on a brave face and I started to wonder again if our love could really go the distance and endure the responsibility of becoming parents so early on in our relationship. Although all of this worry was going on beneath the surface, when we looked at each other, I could just tell that our love was something special. I realised in that moment that this perfect romance had turned into more of a black comedy. I just hoped it would have a happy ending.

An overwhelming sense of loneliness welled up inside me as I looked around the club that night. I was surrounded by all of my closest friends on the dance floor. The same people who, I started to think, may not want to know me in six months time when I was carrying around a nappy bag and my breasts were leaking milk. I knew that they all cared about me but none of them had babies and I really did feel like I was in danger of becoming an outsider. I worried that I might lose a lot of my friends when I inevitably had to become a lot more responsible and maybe, in their eyes, a lot less fun. I lamented to myself that the party girl who used to dance all night on tables would become a distant memory to my friends. I'd be the forgotten girl.

Then my thoughts flipped around and I started to re-evaluate myself. What type of person did I really want to be? Did I really want to be known as a party girl anyway? Then it dawned on me. I really wasn't sure who I was. Making the transition from good-time girl to motherhood was causing me to have a bit of an identity crisis. It made me worry that I might be too unsure of myself to parent a child and help it to establish its place in the world, when I had yet to work out who I wanted to be.

As the night came to a close Gary and I made our excuses and managed to avoid the inevitable after party. We headed straight to bed when we got home, but I couldn't get to sleep for ages. Lying in bed, I started to feel some odd sensations coming from my stomach. I think most of this was just my mind playing tricks on me as I wasn't even 12 weeks but I couldn't help tune in to all the sensations as the bun in my oven continued to bake! At that moment I started to feel a real sense of love for and attachment to this little life that we had created. Eventually I dozed off with a warm fuzzy feeling and had a great sleep. When I woke up the next day, hangover-free, we drove to the hospital for our first scan.

As we sat in the waiting room, I started to feel a little bit paranoid. The room was full of what looked like married couples, and most of them were a lot older than my Gary and me. The critical voices in my head began again as I scanned the room:

"They are looking at me like I shouldn't be here."

"I hope they don't think this is an accident."

These voices turned into worry:

"What if something is wrong with the baby?"

Suddenly a sonographer called me through: "Deirdre – in you come, please."

Gary and I clasped hands as I lay on my back and cold gel was squeezed all over my now ever-so-slightly raised belly. The midwife began her search.

"Here is your baby," she said pointing to an unquestionably human image of a tiny baby that would eventually walk around all by itself and maybe even grow up to have its own children one day. I turned to Gary and saw tears forming in his eyes. He usually cried when he was happy so this was actually a good sign!

"It's coming on fine. I will book your next appointment where we will investigate and do some screening tests to eliminate the possibility of Down syndrome. There's only a slim chance but it's a test that we offer to everyone."

What? I thought to myself.

There appeared to be many gaps in my knowledge of pregnancy. I really hadn't done my homework. I wrote down all my future appointments. There were so many, from vaccines to screenings to antenatal classes. I was already extremely busy with my new job, but it seemed like my life was about to get even busier. I guessed it was all part of the preparation for becoming a mum.

We left the appointment, sharing tears of happiness. We were holding a flimsy black-and-white printout showing the little blob that was our baby. We speculated whether it was going to be a boy or a girl. What would we call it?

The thrill of seeing our baby for the first time was exhilarating. As we made our way home and listened to music blasting from the car speakers, I felt really good. In that precise moment, it felt like we were both driving together into a new and exciting future. It was a beautiful moment. The reality had well and truly set in now, and there was no turning back. The baby was going to be here in a matter of months and I was going to be a mum! When we got home, I went for a lie down on the couch. I could hear Gary rustling around in the kitchen and wondered what he was up to. Suddenly he appeared holding a cake with three lit candles on it and a gift. I unwrapped the gift with great anticipation, hoping that it might be the nice dress I saw last week in Mango. It was and I was delighted with the very thoughtful gesture. He made a joke that for my next gift he would buy me a new comfortable bra, some TENA Ladys in case I sneezed and peed myself and some Bio-Oil to counter the possibility of stretch marks! I realised that Gary was going to see me in a whole new light and encounter some of those very intimate and somewhat embarrassing problems that I would experience. I also remembered that I really needed to do my homework as there was so much I didn't yet know, but first I had a birthday cake to devour – being pregnant was hungry work!

Surprise! I'm Pregnant!

One thing I did actually brush up on was to find out when I should share the news with my family. I found the idea of telling people quite daunting. Who do you tell first? How do you do it? Gary and I were happy with our decision to keep the baby, but this didn't seem to make the idea of telling people any easier. I should have been really excited to share the news with those closest to me, but I was terrified. I wanted them to be happy for me, to say they would support me, to see that Gary and I were in love and that despite the unplanned nature of the pregnancy, we were determined to make it work because it felt right for us. I knew that the news would definitely come as a shock to my family. I had never looked after a baby in my life and now I was going to tell them I was having one of my own! I was sure that their mouths would hit the floor and that they may even laugh uncontrollably at the thought of me saying I wanted to be a mum, considering my history with babies, i.e. I hadn't even looked after one before.

Once again I felt a sense of dread that I would be judged. I was, after all, their little girl and I hadn't exactly done things in the usual order. I wasn't married, I had yet to figure out what I wanted to do with my life and I didn't even own a car, let alone a house. I was worried they would think I was too young to have a baby in today's society. I worried that they would be angry with me, criticise me and call me irresponsible for getting myself up the duff by accident. I got myself into a state of panic about the whole idea of letting the cat, or baby to be more exact, out of the bag. For a moment, I appreciated how nice it had been over the last couple of months, with only Gary and I knowing our little secret. It was now time to let the world know my decision and I was frightened about how it was going to impact on me.

On the long bus journey home from Glasgow to Skye, I ruminated for hours about how to tell them. I considered taking my parents out to a busy restaurant and breaking the news to them over dinner. I hoped that being in a public place surrounded by happy diners might dull their reaction. It seemed foolproof, but then I remembered that I'd have to refuse the pre-dinner drink. This would no doubt blow my cover, as refusing a nice glass of wine was not my usual style, as you know, dear readers! So, instead I waited for the perfect opportunity over my weekend at home and gently broke the news to them in the house when the right opportunity arose.

I arrived home in Skye on a frosty February evening and was welcomed by my long-eared, slobbery-faced basset hound, Millie, at the front door. My mum and dad bought her for me when I was eight years old. Thinking back, I actually looked after her pretty well during my time at home. I suppose you could say she was my first child. Although, much easier to care for and entertain than a human child. I adored Millie and there were times growing up when I could actually say she was my best friend. In her younger days she used to follow me around everywhere and would literally chase me up the stairs, but she had got significantly fatter and lazier in recent years, so I had to tempt her up to my bedroom with some sliced ham so that we could catch up properly. We lay next to each other on my old bed. My bedroom was still filled with pictures of my life so far, my Paulo Coelho quotes, but most of the glow-in-the-dark stars I used to gaze at while falling asleep were either gone or hanging off and the soothing glow from my purple lava lamp was fading. Millie licked my face and I clung on to her tightly, telling her how much I had missed her. I confided in her that day. She was one of my oldest and dearest friends, after all, and I knew that she wouldn't judge me. I practised what I was going to say to my family in a few hours on poor old Millie. She probably didn't really care what I was saying and just wanted more sliced ham but it felt good none the less.

"I have something to tell you, Millie. Your mummy, *me*, is going to be a mummy to somebody else, although this time it's a human. Don't look at me like that with your sad droopy eyes; I've been a good mum to you, so why wouldn't I be to a baby? I know this isn't what you want to hear, but I've made my decision. I'm going to have a baby with that guy you liked the last time I was up. Remember him? The one who took you out for a walk and fed you treats under the table? Yes, I know he is probably too good for me, but he wants this too. Stop looking at me like that. You're not mad, are you? Bark once if you're against this or for ever hold your peace."

I took her paw and placed it on my ever-more protruding bump, which I had managed to disguise under my oversized boyfriend T-shirt. We just lay there, in silence, for hours. She never did bark. I took her silence as a sign that she was with me on this one and had my back. I knew I could always count on Millie.

My family began to return home from work and school, so I headed down to say hello to them, acting as normal as possible. I didn't tell everyone there and then. Instead I waited until after we all had dinner together later that night. Straight after pudding I capitalised on the sugar rush and went for it. For some reason I decided to stand up. Everyone looked over at me awkwardly wondering what I was going to do.

Here goes:

"I have something to tell you all."

My mother, father, three sisters and brother looked at me in a sort of stunned silence, and then my little sister blurted out, "You're up the duff."

I didn't even get to respond before the rest of my family started to join in.

"You've got a role in a new movie?" my other sister interjected.

"You've decided to move back home?" my mother asked.

"You're going back to acting school?" my father added.

"One of you is right." I said.

They all looked around the table at each other, intrigued as to who might have got it right. The attention slowly drifted back towards me and I felt my mouth go a little bit dry and my palms start to sweat. I looked around at my family nervously, smiling at them, trying to find the right words to say. I don't think any of them thought for a second that my little sister was the one who was right. Far from it. In fact, I'm 100 per cent certain that they ruled that one out straight away!

"Er, I... I don't really know how to put this... err."

"C'mon, Deirdre, the suspense is killing us," my brother said.

And in that moment I got over my stage fright and blurted out the words...

"I'm thirteen weeks pregnant."

As forks and mouths began to hit the dinner plates, I could see that there was a look of disbelief and confusion on pretty much everybody's face. I think they thought I was joking and were puzzled as to why there was no punchline yet! My news had effectively silenced one of the noisiest families I know. I said the words again: "I am actually pregnant. I'm having a baby."

My mother, who I'd imagined would be so disappointed and upset, was actually delighted. She held me until I couldn't breathe. She couldn't wait to share this "wonderful news" with her brother, my uncle, who lived in the next house across the field. I was way off the mark in guessing my mother's reaction but my father's reaction was a little more predictable.

"What about your acting career?" he said in a more serious tone than my mother had used when she practically punched the air with joy and exclaimed her happiness seconds earlier. I gave a response that sounded prepared but in fact kind of just rolled off the tip of my tongue.

"Well, Dad, I'm paraphrasing a bit here but Sanford Meisner says that to be an interesting actor, to be an interesting human being even – you first need to be authentic and embrace who you really are. I'm embracing this because I instinctively know it's what I want. Also, look on the bright side. I might be in with a better chance of getting any roles that would benefit from life experience in motherhood."

My dad looked at me with a slight grin now forming on his face. I think he enjoyed my response and could see that I was genuinely happy about becoming a mum.

To my delight, there was no need for police intervention that night. As everyone began to get over the initial shock of my announcement, they began to celebrate. I felt very relieved and happy as I looked around at everyone's now-smiling faces. My sisters would become aunties, my brother would become an uncle, my parents would become grandparents and my uncle would be here to meet the newest addition to our family. It was a poignant and beautiful moment which brought a little bit of light and hope back into the family after a tough couple of months for my stricken uncle. My mother wanted to share her joy with him immediately, so she grabbed me by the arm and off we went across the windy field to tell him the news.

"I'm going to meet the next generation?" My uncle looked me in the eye with so much hope and warmth.

"You sure are, Uncle Iain."

"This is all extremely exciting! You never cease to surprise us all, Deirdre. You two are going to be great parents! Honestly, this is what life is all about, Deirdre, and I am so happy for you both."

My uncle had a few chances to bond with Gary over the few visits we had in Skye up to this point. Gary knew how important he was to me, and that any free hours I had I wanted to be in his company, to hear all his tales of adventures. My uncle knew how important Gary was to me too. He had a way of separating the good from the bad and he always told me how lucky I was to find someone like him, that it was somewhat rare that we had to do our best to stick together.

All my sisters formed around me like a cheerleading group as we sat by the fire with hot chocolate (a sweet change from Prosecco) and talked about how the rest of the world would take the news, all of us trying to adjust to the news that the second youngest in the family was going to give birth, change nappies, potty train and breastfeed by the time the youngest had left school. It was a weird and wonderful evening. It was the first time in thirteen weeks that I really felt that I could do it. I couldn't believe how much energy I wasted being terrified of telling the people who care about me the most. I called Gary to tell him that everyone took the news better than I had expected and that now it was time to tell his side of the family. We were continuing our game of chess.

It wasn't long until the reality of my pregnancy set back in. My mother delivered breakfast to me in bed the following morning along with many hand-picked pregnancy books. I started to flick through the books one by one and became extremely insecure. The books were filled with women and their perfect breasts, bumps and babies. Was I really up to this? Was I ready? Why was there no one my age telling me it's going to be fine? Reality had sunk in and there was nowhere to run. There were so many hurdles to overcome and one way or another I was going to have to pull myself out of this state of mind and settle into my own journey, as each day brought new changes and growth.

Knowing Me, Knowing You

It was now time to tell Gary's family of our destiny and we did so face-to-face during a week they returned to Scotland from Abu Dhabi in late February. Having not long imparted the news to my parents, it was time to do it all again with Gary's. Of course, being the tactful, caring couple we were, we decided to collect a curry from their favourite Indian restaurant, the Shish Mahal in Glasgow, to give them that warm and fuzzy feeling as we settled in for a night by the television.

That night, I kept nudging Gary with my feet as he sat at the opposite end of the sofa, as a way of letting him know *I think the time is right*. The suspense was killing me. I was filled with concerns that they would think that I was putting their son's life on hold, that they would think we were rushing into this too quickly, that we weren't ready to be parents of their first grandchild. I knew that I had made a good impression on them and we had a chance to bond on our recent holiday, but still, how would they react?

"Deirdre and I are having a baby," Gary revealed to the room.

After a few delayed seconds, the surprise wore off and we were surrounded by warm hugs and kisses. It really was as easy as that. I felt a rush of relief and wished I hadn't worried so much about their response. After all, they knew we shared the most important ingredient to becoming parents. *Love*.

I was made to feel like the daughter that his parents had

never had. They took me under their wings. I had won the jackpot. They really were happy that I was going to give them their first grandchild and they were so ready for it.

I was now living with them in their house, which Gary was looking after while they were away, although we continued to hunt for a place to call our own before the baby got here. It was lovely to have the chance to get to know his parents even better. They knew all about the uncertainty I felt, having been in a similar position when they had welcomed their first son into the world when they were a young couple in love. I had finally found another young mum who I could talk to, albeit with more than twenty years between us and our experiences. It dawned on me that each generation feels exactly the same way when faced with young pregnancy and are scared and vulnerable. I thought about how lucky I was to be giving birth at a time when our health services were so advanced, a time when workplaces were obliged to offer maternity pay, a time when I had options for pain relief during labour, a time when it was OK for your boyfriend to be by your side all day.

"What was it like to give birth back then?" I quizzed Gary's mum, hoping for a simple answer.

"I had a fourteen-hour labour with my first. I remained in hospital for eight days before bringing him home. At night, I remember a massive cockroach would creep along the ward floor, going under one bed to the other. Once, I rang for the nurse but no one came so I lifted him into bed with me (which was not allowed) and tucked us both under the covers so tightly in case the cockroach came for us. With Gary, my labour was slightly more uncomfortable as he was eleven days late. I got induced with Gary, which was so upsetting because I wanted to go myself. I cried all the way to the hospital after I received home-made dumpling to wish me all the best from neighbours.

I was woken up by the girl in the next bed to me telling me I had been groaning all night; I must have fallen asleep because of the sleeping pill they had given me. I was definitely in labour when I was woken up by her at 3am, and three hours later Gary was born."

In that moment I realised, for possibly the first time, that I too was actually going to have to *give birth*. Labour really didn't seem as straightforward as it looked on *Scrubs*. But she was still here to tell the tale, so it couldn't be that bad, could it? I'd got a lot to learn.

The initial tiredness of the first trimester was fading away and I spent my whole working week trying to keep up with my job in the city, hiding myself under baggy clothing and keeping the morning sickness at bay by eating ginger snaps and dashing out for fresh air pretending to be on a cigarette break. I got the impression that many of my new work colleagues thought I was odd as I declined drinks after work (and sometimes during lunch); however, I took great comfort in the fact that they didn't know the *'real'* me and that they must think I was just a very mature, wise, career-hungry nineteen-year-old making her way in the world, which was, to be fair, a hilarious thought. Most of my office hours, between ruining people's days on the telephone trying to collect debt and navigating my way through many possible fraud transactions, were now spent thinking about the baby and everything I would have to put in place before the baby entered the world.

Temporary

I had surrounded myself with a lot of temporary souls in my city life. People who would know me only superficially, who craved to be around my wild spirit, who like wolves would appear with the nightfall and howl at the moon. And back home, I had left behind my few true friends, who were still figuring out what life they were going to carve out for themselves. It hit home that the next step on my journey was releasing my secret to my friends and I wondered what the response would be.

I had not long escaped one of the places that made me feel most vulnerable – school. Now judgement day was looming and I felt as though I was back in the school playground waiting for the comments to come. It felt like everything I had worked so hard to run away from was coming at me full force. The thought of being judged, spoken about behind my back, being the butt of everyone's jokes, filled me with dread. I thought I'd left all that behind the day I left for Glasgow.

Something that shone through quickly once I began to impart the news to those friends closest to me was the value of true friendship. I realised quickly that the girl who stays up with you all night and passes you tissues as you cry over a break-up really does care about you. I decided to test the water with my friend Sadie, who I trusted to be honest with me. It was a conversation I needed to have, with someone who knew all of me. Our friendship had blossomed after a bitching match over who was going to get what part in our acting class, and developed into us spending every hour under the sun together. This is what you call real, deep, no-holds-barred friendship. We knew each other inside out. There were no secrets up until now, apart from the baby. I knew she was the perfect person to impart this truth bomb on. She was going to question me like no one else would dare.

"I'm pregnant."

"Jesus Christ, I don't know what to say," she replied.

We spoke for hours about everything that was going through my mind, reflecting on how my life was going to change. For ever.

"What did your parents say?" Sadie asked.

"They were kind of accepting of it. I felt quite awkward talking to them about it."

"Were you pretending to be drunk last week at your birthday?"

"Yes, I was completely sober."

"Actually, I think you're going to make it as an actress because I didn't know."

"Very funny."

"What does Gary think?'

"He's excited, he thinks I'm going to look hot pregnant."

"Eh, you're going to look really weird. How will your skin manage to stretch that far?"

"I'm already putting on Bio-Oil; apparently it helps with stretch marks."

"I genuinely don't know if you're going to fit a baby in there. You're going to have to feed it more than Pot Noodles and Pop Tarts."

"I've got a grown-up job actually – so I might upgrade my diet to real food."

"Good luck with that, babe. Can he cook?"

"Yes, he makes some really good meals. It's going to be fine."

"Fine?"

"Yes, I think everything is going to be fine."

"Where are you going to live?"

"Well, we can stay here at his parents until we find our own place. We have started looking and hopefully will get something before the baby arrives."

"OK, so what about acting? Have you not got that big audition coming up?"

"I'm just going to call them and say I can't do it any more. I'll be back on stage in eleven months, I'm sure of it."

"We'll see…"

"That's not very positive."

"I'm still in shock that's all. I need a bottle of wine. Can you drink wine at all?"

"Apparently you can have the odd one. It can help to 'de-stress' you."

"God, I need more than one to de-stress me. What are you going to call it?"

"No idea yet. I don't know if it's going to be a boy or a girl."

"If it's a girl, you can call her Sadie, OK?"

"I don't want to name my baby after someone who jumped off a table playing air guitar and broke their ankle at my birthday."

"The floor was wet."

"Babe, you've got to stop jumping off tables when you're drunk."

"Are you showing yet?"

"No, nothing really, maybe a little. I'm just feeling really tired all the time."

"You always say you're tired."

"No, I mean really tired, like waking up wishing it was bedtime."

"Do you have morning sickness?"

"I had one bout of morning sickness but that was it. I'm so worried about how different my body is going to be. I am just coming up to finishing my first trimester, time is passing so quickly."

"I'm actually coming round to seeing the funny side of it. You being pregnant."

"Is there a funny side?"

"Yes, babe, and if anyone is going to get through this, it's you."

As I gained some confidence from our conversation, I knew that I would have at least one friend sticking by me and so I began to share the news with my wider connections and sat back as replies came in saying something like this:

Well, I guess congratulations are in order. Last time I saw you, you were walking home in your Halloween costume three nights after Halloween with a sausage supper. There's always room for improvement.

This is the earliest April Fool you have ever done, I am definitely not falling for this one.

Start filming now, this is going to be Oscar worthy. Good luck and all that.

Oh that's so lovely, you're going to make a great mum. LOL.

I'm too hung-over for your jokes right now.

Is Donald Trump the father?

The First Trimester:

A summary of what's happening to you and your baby & the things I wish I had known

Pregnancy usually lasts around nine months or forty weeks. Pregnancy is broken into three periods called 'trimesters'. Each trimester lasts around thirteen weeks. The first thirteen weeks of pregnancy is known as your first trimester. The next thirteen is called the second trimester and the last thirteen, you guessed it, is called the third trimester! Here's some advice to get you through the first one.

OMG, I'm Pregnant! What Do I Do Now?

You can buy a pregnancy test from your local pharmacy, or pick one up from your GP practice or local midwife. Some pregnancy tests can confirm your pregnancy up to 6 days before your missed period (which is 5 days before your expected period) but each pregnancy test will come with its own instructions and time frames. After you have taken the pregnancy test that confirms you're pregnant, it's time to start thinking about everything you need to do from now on to make sure you're doing what's best for you and your baby. You may have guessed it, but I really did know *nothing* about pregnancy, or exactly what was happening to me, or what I should be doing to ensure I was on the right track, so here is my advice to you, to help you get through your first trimester!

Taking baby steps...

- Book an appointment with your local midwife. You may feel, like me, that your GP is the obvious choice but it's not. Your local GP practice can put you straight in contact with your midwife as can your local family centre to avoid even more appointments!
- Start a prenatal vitamin (more about that later...).
- Speak to your partner about how you are going to share the news with family – most people wait until the end of the first trimester to tell family, when the chance of a miscarriage is lower. However, this can be so difficult as you're most likely to be feeling the symptoms of pregnancy – tiredness, sickness and emotional at this stage – the time when you need family support and care. It isn't medically important to tell family – it is a personal decision. Talk it through with your partner – do what feels right for you.
- Ideally, developing a healthy lifestyle comes before pregnancy but as many pregnancies are unplanned it is important to stop smoking, taking drugs, drinking alcohol, etc immediately – if you are on prescription medication speak to your doctor to ensure it is safe to continue.
- Educate yourself by finding out about your local services – ask your midwife for information on support groups, classes and/or useful books to read.

Once you have met your midwife, your pregnancy care journey will really begin. You will be asked to give personal health details, as well as insights into your family's health history. This is to identify any complex histories that may impact on your or your baby's health and well-being during the pregnancy and beyond. Ask any questions during these conversations – check up with your family for any history that might be relevant. You may also be asked to go through a physical exam which would involve possible weight measurement and height for Body Mass Index calculations, blood pressure, urine check – to get baseline measurements. From this point on your diary will begin to fill up with further testing and screening test options available to you. It's important that you make the decisions that you want and therefore important to get as much information as possible before making a decision about screening tests and so on.

Body changes

There will be few changes to your body at this stage; the best is yet to come! Your baby is still quite small and although it develops faster in the first trimester than any other time during pregnancy you may only begin to see a small bump appear as you reach the end of this period. Weight gain during pregnancy is something we all fear and, yes, moving into the second trimester you need to make sure you are eating enough for all the work your body is doing to create mini-you. I'm going to burst a myth for you: you do not have to eat for two during pregnancy. Pregnancy isn't an excuse to add any extra calories to your diet; as you move into the third trimester it is recommended to only add an extra 200 calories a day but at this stage a balanced diet and regular exercise is key. Did you know that eating well during pregnancy can reduce your child's risk of having heart disease or diabetes in later life? If that's not a good reason to fill yourself up with goodness I don't know what is!

What the hell is happening to my breasts?

Most women who become pregnant notice changes in their breasts. I know I certainly did. During the first trimester, at around five weeks, I noticed that my breasts had become tender. For instance, a light bump on the train to work was sore! My breasts also started to grow – which was an added bonus for my boyfriend who noticed even before I did! Hormonal changes during pregnancy cause increased blood flow and changes in the breast tissue. This in turn can make your breasts feel tender, swollen, more sensitive to touch and sometimes a little bit tingly. If I was to describe how it was for me, I'd say that it's like a slightly exaggerated version of how my breasts feel before my period arrives. As pregnancy progresses there can be a number of noticeable breast changes, which are good to know about in advance, and will be covered later in the book.

What is morning sickness really?

You're probably not surprised to hear that nausea and vomiting are quite common in pregnancy. In fact, around 80 per cent of women experience nausea and/or vomiting in the first twelve weeks of pregnancy. This is yet another bonus symptom of pregnancy that you can blame on hormonal changes, according to the medical books. The one thing the medical books get wrong, however, is using the term morning sickness, as the nausea and/or vomiting can strike at any time of the day or night and can sometimes last all day. I once had to vomit out of the window of a moving car – not ideal! The vomiting is usually quite predictable and you usually get plenty of warning as to when you're actually going to be sick. I just happened to be in my boyfriend's car on the motorway and couldn't stop it from happening. Although morning sickness is unpleasant, it doesn't put your baby at any increased risk and should usually clear up during the second trimester. If you have any concerns about your morning sickness and you are not eating, unable to keep down fluids, feeling unwell, have a temperature, etc contact your midwife.

Morning sickness will make you feel like you have taken one too many tequila shots. You'll not have missed this feeling, so here are some tips to get you through it!

- Stock up on ginger biscuits (or anything that contains ginger – it was my magic potion).
- Eat smaller meals more often during the day – carry snacks.
- Tiredness can make you feel more sick, so take rests when you can.
- Place yourself next to a toilet at work. At times it can come on very quickly!
- Take a fan to work with you, or take regular breaks to walk outside in the fresh air.
- Don't be adventurous with your foods – stick to the food you like.
- Drink more water, or ginger tea, keep to fluids that will be gentle on your stomach.
- Eat a good breakfast that is rich in fibre (am I beginning to sound like your mother yet?).

Is it time for bed yet?

Tiredness can be another early sign that you have a bun in the oven, and it is a feeling that will be very present in the first trimester, and well, forever. It's natural to feel tiredness during pregnancy; after all, your body is working hard to create a baby! I used to love falling asleep on the train to my city job, or having the excuse of sneaking up to my bedroom for a nap.

- Keep hydrated – carry a water bottle with you, jazz it up with some lemon or sliced strawberries!
- Spend as much time as you can out in the fresh air during breaks at work, taking evening strolls – this might come as a surprise but exercising might actually make you feel less tired!
- Ask for help – yes, us ladies find this hard sometimes, but reach out to your boyfriend and get him to man up and stick the kettle on.
- Try and get a full night's sleep. Go to bed earlier and get the recommended eight hours in and fit in some rests while you can.
- Have a look to see if you have any pregnancy fitness classes in the area; yoga and swimming are two forms of recommended exercise.
- Make sure you are taking good prenatal vitamins and are getting a balance of nutrients – ask your local nutrition store for ones related to pregnancy so you can ensure you are stocked up on your nutritional needs to avoid tiredness and fatigue!
- Keep an eye on your iron levels; you can get iron through eating dark green vegetables such as kale or spinach.
- Make sure you have a balanced diet with nutrients that should provide you with more energy.
- Take some nice long baths, play a chill-out album, read books and make yourself a priority.
- Carry some light snacks that will provide you with energy – such as a banana.

Emotions and emotional health

You may feel overwhelmed with emotion, feeling like you're watching the end of *La La Land* on repeat. Your hormones will be all over the place in the first trimester as your body adapts to the developing baby, so please feel free to have a good old cry into your bowl of soup, it's the new normal for you. Surprise, joy, anger, fear, love, sadness are just some of the emotions you may feel during pregnancy and although some will be more difficult than others to deal with, it is *so* normal to feel emotional.

- You may feel consumed with worry at night, leaving you with sleepless nights – try simple breathing exercises which will bring you back to you and calm you down.
- You may feel like you're not ready to become a mum. But don't judge yourself based on what society says; your situation is unique to you and what you want.
- Talk openly to your support network and come up with strategies to help when you become overwhelmed with emotion, remembering, always, that it is natural.
- If you feel your emotions are out of control, contact your midwife. Hormones can affect everyone differently.
- Mood swings can often creep up on you – one day you are up, the next you are down. We often hear about post-natal depression, but many women can also experience depression during pregnancy. You should not feel ashamed, as it's very common and can usually be explained by hormone changes. So make sure you are looking after you, and book an appointment with your doctor.

Sharing the news

I was really nervous about how my parents would react: I feared they would be disappointed in me or even angry that I was throwing away the career I had spent so long trying to establish, or think I was just too young to be a parent. But in the end, they were so supportive and gave me all the love and advice I needed. Not everyone is so lucky. Telling your parents that you're pregnant can feel awkward, especially if you aren't sure how they're going to react. Even if you're worried that your parents are going to have a negative reaction to the news, it's a good idea to tell them sooner rather than later. It's also a good idea to plan ahead how and where you're going to tell them.

- Decide whether you want to reveal the news in private, such as at a family meal or one-on-one, or reveal the news while out and about in public. There are advantages and disadvantages to both. For instance, announcing it while out in public can lessen immediate negative reactions simply by virtue of the presence of other people.
- Having someone there to act as moral support, such as a friend, sibling, partner or even a doctor, when you tell parents can make the conversation easier.
- You might find it easier to introduce the discussion when doing something together, like a household chore or when walking the dog. Doing a task together can help make telling them feel less overwhelming.
- Stay calm when you tell them and let them know how much you need/want their support.

Just remember: there are plenty of people in your life, as well as organisations out there specifically set up for this type of situation, that can provide you with all the support you need, if you don't get it from your family. For example:

- www.tommys.org – Tommy's is a great resource at all stages of your pregnancy, to help you grow your understanding of how to have a healthy pregnancy and to answer any concerns you may have. They also have great tips on how to speak out about your pregnancy and where to find further support.
- www.themix.org.uk/sex-and-relationships/pregnancy-and-parenthood – The Mix offers a wide range of support to under-25 mums-to-be – not only do they provide a free phone service for you to call if you need to talk, but they also have great information and relatable forums for you to join.

Looking back, I wish I hadn't spent so many hours worrying about how I was going to break the news. That I hadn't created an image of myself in my mind that I was not ready, that I was too young and it wasn't the right time, that I needed to have a good job, that my life needed to be perfect. I realise now that, even if I had created the perfect life, life has a way of always throwing surprises at you. So when the unexpected happens, remember that no matter how it might feel initially, you are not alone and reaching out to friends and family is always a good idea. In fact, keeping your head healthy is a pregnancy must in itself.

- Build support around you. This might be with the father of your child, or your best friend, or your parents. Share your feelings with others. It's better out than in, as they say.
- If you have worries, or lack of support from family around, reach out to your midwife and other organisations set up to help young mothers. They can help open doors

to further support networks to help you deal with the reality of your pregnancy.

- Remember that millions of women and couples have been in your position, you are not alone.
- STOP being so hard on yourself – you are not irresponsible. I think everything happens for a reason, you just need to know that your fate isn't what you always plan it to be and sometimes you just need to trust in yourself and know that you'll get through it.
- This baby is yours. You are responsible for it, no one else. Take pride in the decisions you make.

Diet and Nutrition

You may have learned something else about me – I'm no chef. But this doesn't make it any less important to make sure that baby and you are getting all the nutrients to stay healthy. So here are some tips on how to keep you on the right track.

Prenatal vitamins

If you're actively trying to conceive, then it is recommended that you start taking folic acid and eat more foods containing folate such as leafy green vegetables, citrus fruits and beans. If your pregnancy was unplanned, then you should start taking folic acid and increase folate intake as soon as you find out you're pregnant. The reason why it is a very important nutrient during pregnancy is because it can help prevent spina bifida. The recommended dose is 0.4mg of folic acid every day before you get pregnant right up to week twelve or the end of the first trimester.

Foods to avoid

Cheese and dairy
Due to bacteria such as listeria, some cheeses are off limits. To be honest, if I'd known in advance that I had to avoid Brie during pregnancy, I may have got myself sterilised when I turned eighteen. It's one of my favourite treats, especially with a bit of cranberry sauce. Alas, I couldn't use the cranberry sauce for my toast and pâté either, as pâté's off the pregnancy menu too as it contains high levels of vitamin A which can be harmful to your growing baby. You can still eat cooked meats though so the cranberry sauce will still come in handy with some turkey at Christmas.

Fortunately, harder cheeses such as Cheddar and Parmesan are usually safe. Softer cheeses made with pasteurised milk are also permitted; this includes cheeses such as cottage cheese and mozzarella. Processed cheeses such as cheese spreads are also OK, so don't throw away your Dairylea just yet! You also want to make sure you are only drinking pasteurised milk and making sure that your sneaky ice cream is made from pasteurised milk too!

Raw or partially cooked eggs
Like your eggs hard boiled? You're in luck! Well-cooked eggs are OK to eat. Just don't be hoping for some sunny-side up runny eggs with your English breakfast while pregnant. Uncooked and raw eggs can contain salmonella, which can cause food poisoning, which is obviously not good if you're pregnant. So make sure you read labels to ensure there are no raw or uncooked eggs in the ingredients.

Raw or undercooked meats
Say bye-bye to your medium-cooked fillet. Yes, all meat and poultry needs to be cooked thoroughly while you are pregnant. This includes sausages, burgers and mince. You need to ensure that all meat is piping hot with no traces of pink or blood. Also, hold the cold meats, as Parma ham, chorizo and salami are all to be avoided too. Always check food labels and ask for information about dishes in restaurants if you are unsure.

Some types of fish and shellfish
Mercury can be found in some fish, which can be dangerous for the development of your baby's nervous system. Limit yourself to no more than two portions of oily fish a week and completely avoid shark (because we all eat so much of it), swordfish and raw shellfish. Raw shellfish can contain harmful bacteria and viruses, so no oysters or caviar, dahling!

Caffeine
I have some even worse news for you: say goodbye to your caffeine hit. Too much caffeine in pregnancy can lead to low birth weight and can also increase the risk of miscarriage. So reduce your daily trips to Starbucks. Your baby will be able to swallow soon and I doubt it will be crying out for an Americano! Limit your caffeine to no more than 200mg a day (two small cups of filter coffee) but remember, caffeine is also found in tea, chocolate, fizzy drinks and energy drinks, so make sure you are making switches to water, herbal teas or decaffeinated coffee.

Foods to seek out

So, as you can see, you are going to have to adjust your diet slightly and avoid certain foods but the good news is there are lots of foods you still can eat, and you want to make sure you include the following foods in your new diet plan.

- At least five portions of fruit and vegetables a day.
- Foods that are high in carbohydrates to give you energy, including pasta, breads and potatoes.
- Protein-rich foods like tofu, beans and lean meats, including chicken, turkey and white fish.
- At least two portions of healthy fatty acids per week, such as found in nuts, avocados and 'oily' fish like salmon or mackerel, which are important for the physical and mental growth of baby!

There you have it, some information on what foods to avoid/ stock up on. I always found it helpful to print food lists out and stick them to my fridge. Keeping your fridge stocked up with the right foods will help you keep on track and it will also help when hunger strikes so you can avoid dipping into the sweetie drawer!

Let's Talk about SEX!

Have I mentioned the word overwhelmed yet? Yes, thought so. You may spend a lot of time worrying about yourself, how everything is going to change, how your body is slowly but surely forgetting its youthful frame, but there is something you might be forgetting about. Yes, *him*, the guy that got you to this book. Remember that thing that got you into this position in the first place? Yes, *sex*! Well, I have some good news for you: sex has got the green light unless otherwise advised by your midwife. I know, I know, you might be insecure of what is happening in your body, you're worried that the baby might feel something, or hear you orgasm, but sex is as important as it always was.

- Your baby is tucked away in its amniotic sac inside the uterus, so it is well away from penetration.
- Sex is wonderful – give yourself the chance to escape your busy head by getting busy and get some pleasure.
- You may need to start getting creative with your positions; as your bump develops it might begin to feel uncomfortable in certain ones!
- If you don't feel like having sex, that's OK, but remember him, and spend some quality time together when you can.

Employment: Know Your Rights!

If you have a job, it's time to have another look over your contract. It should spell out the legal rights to which you are entitled, including being allowed paid time off for your antenatal care, any maternity leave, maternity pay or allowance and your protections against unfair treatment, discrimination or dismissal.

- Each employer may have different set terms, but make sure you know the ins and outs of your own rights.
- Tell your employer before turning fifteen weeks pregnant – if you find out after fifteen weeks, let them know as soon as possible. The sooner you let your work know the quicker support can be put into place and a discussion can be opened up so that you can plan ahead.
- Make sure your partner also informs his work, as he ought to be entitled to some paternity leave.
- If you don't have a job, make sure to talk to your midwife about what you may be entitled to.

Baby Budget

Yes, I know we are only in the first trimester, but guess what... babies can be expensive! Whether or not you are in a job that will pay you maternity leave, the income in your household is going down, so spending some time getting your finances in order is time well spent. Every motherhood shop in the Amazon jungle has their eyes on you – so here are some tips, to navigate your way through it!

- Find out what benefits you are entitled to and what financial help you can receive in your local area.
- Loyalty cards can help you save money in the long run.
- It's never too early to stock up on deals of washing powder, nappies, wipes, etc – you will use it all!
- Sharing is caring – welcome any hand-me-downs, gifts, unused baby bottles – babies are expensive, welcome the support!
- Shop around for the best deals. Don't just buy the shiny new pram or changing mat because it looks so good in the shop window. The Internet can be wonderful for bargain hunters, as are charity shops!
- Look ahead and prepare a finance list to evaluate where you are, what money is expected to come in and when. Once baby is here, the last thing on your mind will be if there is enough money in your account for your electricity bill!
- Set budgets – not as an individual, but as a household. Have an understanding of who is paying what, when so there is no need for awkward situations to arise, teamwork is key!

When to See a Doctor

Here are some signs to look out for that may indicate you need to seek medical advice promptly in the first trimester.

- Heavy vaginal bleeding (spotting can be common but if this worsens see your GP)
- Severe abdominal pain
- Pain when urinating
- High temperature
- Feeling very thirsty suddenly

Your Baby's Growth in the First Trimester

The length of your pregnancy is calculated from the first day of your last period. How do you like your eggs in the morning? Well, seeing as you're reading this book, I'll take it the answer was fertilised! As a result, a new life is starting to form inside of you, congratulations! Knowing that a baby is growing inside you is astonishing; pregnancy is an incredible process and it still blows my mind that our bodies know how to do all this without us even consciously thinking about it!

Weeks 1–4

As the fertilised egg grows into an embryo, a watertight membrane known as the amniotic sac begins to form around it. This sac gradually fills with fluid to help protect and cushion the embryo during pregnancy. Other fun things that are happening include the growth of the placenta, also known as the afterbirth! I have to say I prefer the name placenta! Sounds much nicer, like it should be an island off the coast of Spain or something!

Weeks 5–8

Your baby is developing nicely and is now about the size of a kidney bean and guess what, it's already moving! You won't feel it at this stage though as the foetus is only about 1 inch long and about one-third of it is the head. You can just about make out the beginnings of a face, body, arms, legs and cute little webbed fingers.

Weeks 9–12

Would you believe me if I told you that your little baby now has identifiable fingers and toes? It can also open and close its hands and mouth. Not only that, you may want to call the beautician and dentist already as fingernails, toenails and teeth have begun to form. Although hands and feet can be easily identified at this stage, it's still a little early to tell your baby's sex via ultrasound. Your baby is around 6cm long at this point.

Shopping List for the First Trimester

- Support bras (the cotton kind) – give your tits the support they deserve! There are some pretty sexy ones out there these days!
- A calendar – you will have lots of scan and screening appointments to remember.
- Ease your stretching skin and smooth any dry parts by investing in some moisturiser to make you feel good.
- Lycra pants (and a few of them!).
- Electric fan – pregnancy can make you feel very warm at times so always good to have something to cool you down.
- Pregnancy diary – wouldn't it be sweet to remember all of this?

- Pregnancy pillow – you'll thank me for it later.
- A good camera (or a camera phone...). Start taking pictures of the development of your bump – it will go on to surprise you!
- Healthy food – keep your fridge stocked up on food to keep you and baby happy and healthy.

Remember: *you* are incredible, what happens through your pregnancy journey is AMAZING. Everything will feel as if it has been put on automatic as the baby develops each day inside of you. Every pregnancy brings with it anxiety and worries but don't let them overwhelm you. You can eat all the best foods, stick to daily exercise, turn up to all your appointments on time, but the one thing you really do need to look after is you and your mind, so always remember to reach out if you need support.

Reflections

We based our decision on having a baby on the love we shared. We didn't have all of the materialistic things in life that one may assume you need to have in order before trying for a baby. We hadn't even had a conversation about having one. I held a lot of fear inside me when I found out about the pregnancy at first, but it diminished immediately once I opened up and told Gary. In fact, when I looked at him after coming out of the bathroom on that cold December day, I blurted out the words, 'We're having a baby' not 'I'm so sorry, I got pregnant.' Everything from within just felt right. It could have only been down to love.

I think love really got me through the ordeal of telling people too. Because although I knew that people may judge me harshly, I knew that I had a handful of people who really loved me. I knew people were going to think something along the lines of *That's not very responsible, becoming a parent when you're just a baby yourself*, but in my heart I knew the life we could give to our baby would be a life full of love. We felt that love was enough.

I'd grown up a lot since leaving home and in the many summers spent away from my parents pursuing my hobbies. I knew deep down that although I may appear irresponsible and selfish at times (because well, I was nineteen remember!) that I had grown up quite a bit by learning the hard way. I was constantly facing my fears, and facing knock-backs in my life. Whether it was rejection letters from acting schools, being told I was too small to play roles or not blonde enough to play the 'pretty' one, acting certainly wasn't the easiest career I could have picked but it had taught me a lot in the years of doing it. It toughened me up a little. It forced me to be adventurous

and it gave me a little taste of freedom from myself. I always enjoyed stepping into the shoes of someone not me. I gained more appreciation that although we all walk around in these beautifully formed bodies, we are all very different. We are all our own characters. We all have our own shit going on that no one on the outside world ever has to know about. But pregnancy wasn't a mask I could hide behind.

I found myself putting some of my acting skills into practice during pregnancy. Whether it was smiling lovingly as people commented on my growing bump, turning up to the office pretending not to be pregnant, or maybe it was just the simple fact that I was pretending to be coping well when sometimes I just wanted everything to stop. I carried on. I was really nailing this new character that I decided to walk in the shoes of and my acting at times was sublime! I really was becoming a new version of me, one that was learning to become a mother.

The odds were stacked against us in the beginning. No one knew what the outcome would be. There are so many who decide to have their children when they least expect it, and when you least expect it sometimes you will just have to trust your heart. Whether you are going to have to bring your baby up alone or you have to go through a pregnancy without support, if you believe it's right in your heart, then you are bound to make it work. It really could have gone either way for me. I had taken a major risk. But I had been taking risks all my life. I'd galloped around arenas horse jumping over fences four times bigger than me. I'd been left stranded on a rock in a surging river. I've dangled into a skip upside down to recover a misplaced item. I risked my reputation wearing the biggest beard as the smallest dwarf in *Snow White and the Seven Dwarfs* school pantomime. I ran away to set up home by the river at

nine years old. I had fallen asleep in my flat too inebriated to close the door, only to be awoken by the postman dropping letters on my head.

Susan Jeffers summed up my feelings perfectly when she wrote the book *Feel the Fear and Do It Anyway*. Did I really need approval from anybody if I knew that I could go through with it? I realised I didn't. I was trusting my instincts. Was I unsure? Yes. Was I terrified? Yes. Did I know what my life was going to look like a year from now? No. But I was facing my fears and doing it anyway. I felt that this was the right thing to do. This was a risk I was gladly willing to take for love.

Just like with my career and at times throughout my life there was one word that I kept referring back to during my pregnancy: *patience*. Patience with my body. Patience with my mind. Patience with people.

It seemed to keep me grounded as many changes began to happen around me. I knew I had to be patient, especially with all the millions of thoughts flying around in my busy mind. Being patient with myself and my feelings enabled me to slow right down and take moments out of my day to re-evaluate, ask myself if I needed a break, or if I just needed a moment to stop. Sometimes you just need to stop. The beauty of pregnancy is that you don't have to do very much as your baby grows inside you, so you'll find moments when you can just be calm. Things begin to settle down after all the highs and lows of the first trimester, and reality settles in that your body is doing something incredible for you. But have patience with your body, mind and people. You deserve to carry that word with you.

PART 2

The Second Trimester

Letting the Dust Settle

A certain unexpected magic happens when you share the news of an expected baby. It really isn't as bad as it all appears to be in your head. Support was something that I had always shunned in the past. I had wanted to be a really independent woman – the one that Beyoncé sings about.

But support was something I would need to welcome in now, at a time in my life that I didn't know what was happening from one second to the next. Everything was speeding up and I still had a suspicion that I was possibly spoken about behind my back, that people were in fact nervous for me, for us. That although we were putting on brave faces, people could still sense that Gary and I were unsure what to make of it all, that we too were nervous. All I heard from everybody was how exciting this was and how wonderful it was to have the first new baby in the family. But we had hit our families, and our friends, with a ton of bricks. I kept hearing those nagging voices in my head.

"Oh my god, I can't believe she got pregnant, what a shame."

"What are we going to do with her?"

"She doesn't even have a real job."

"I think she wants to be an actress, this is going to kill her career."

Many friends were beginning to take longer to return text messages and the invitation to nights out lessened. As the news settled in as 'fact', many of my temporary friends fell completely off the radar. I knew that most of them couldn't relate to what I was going through, and why should they? They had their whole lives to look forward to and I wasn't going to get in the way of that. I continued to love them all for passing through my life and giving me many memories to cherish, but I knew that I needed to build a support network of people who really cared, who wanted to care. Who were willing to grow with me on this journey even though it was so different to theirs. I quickly realised that my mum had been right all along – you can count all your close friends on one hand and here was me, thinking it was so important and cool to have so many.

I knew our families were there for us both, and that they would support us. I don't think I ever realised how much I relied upon them until then. I'd spent the previous few years doing it my way, and now all I wanted was for all my sisters and my brother to rally round me and help me navigate my way through pregnancy and beyond. During the past four years we had been brought closer together by the news that we were going to lose our uncle and now I wondered if they felt that they were going to lose me too as I crossed over into the role of mother. We had only ever needed each other throughout childhood and now we were all growing up, separating, becoming our own people in the world. I had been the first to flee the nest.

I wished I was able to fly back to them all and ask them for one last chance to build mud huts with them in the surrounding moor, peel prawns with them until our hands bled, have water fights into the dusk, swim in the Fairy Pools, set up flower shops for tourists, argue over clothes, come up with plans to get our babysitters fired so our mum and dad could come home from work. I wanted to experience it all again, as their second youngest sister, not the one who is becoming a mum. I used to thrive in the mischief that went on; we enjoyed the possibility of getting into a little bit of trouble, as long as there was a way out. I didn't know the way out of this one. It was as if it was meant to end up this way.

One of my biggest concerns now, having shared the news to everyone, was my younger sister, Clare. She was just about to sit her exams in high school and in a matter of months she was going to morph into a new role as aunt. I worried what people were saying to her at school and how she felt when people asked her if her sister was actually pregnant. How did she answer that question? She was the most precious of them all, she was my little sister. The most beautiful little girl you could cast your eyes on, I always wanted to protect her, to preserve her innocence before she ventured out into the big bad world.

I can remember the day she took me aside in the playground in primary school to tell me that her teacher had asked everyone to stand up in the classroom and speak about someone they admired.

"I picked you," she said with her curly blonde locks, blue eyes and innocent face, aged eight. I wondered how differently she must have felt about me now. The pressure on her to grow up and face the world was enough for her, without me getting all the attention and support from everyone. She was a flower ready to blossom, in her own time, at her own pace, and I was eager not to let her down.

These sorts of thoughts and anxieties would lessen over time and the more I began to focus on the joy that I was bringing to people's lives the less I worried that they were only being compassionate because they felt sorry for our situation. Every day something else would arrive by post. Tiny newborn clothes, a hand-me-down cradle and nursing chair from my cousin down south, letters from aunts reaching out to me and letting me know they were there, and all sorts of treats for me and baby. Even our weekly shopping trips to the supermarket would finish with the trolley being packed to the gunnels with nappies, baby wipes and bibs found on the deals lane, perched on top of our groceries. We couldn't resist! This baby was on its way and we had to be ready.

Time to Get Responsible

As we continued on our journey to get ready for baby's arrival, I knew that I still had a lot of growing up to do. One of the first priorities was to find a place for us all to live. We had many conversations about where we wanted to make our first home together. We were unsure whether we wanted to live in the city or remain in the country, but in the end we decided the most important factor was for our home to be within washing, I mean *walking* distance from grandparents. If I was sure of anything at this point, I was sure we were going to need support and to our delight a small, repossessed house came on to the market just two streets away from Gary's parents. This house needed everything done to it from new paint, new toilets and new flooring, but it was perfect for us. We now had five months to go until the baby was due – that would be enough time to get our new home ready, right?

There was suddenly a lot more on our to-do list. The list was getting bigger by the day and although there were many items that could be easily ticked off, there were many improvements that I would also need to make, within myself, to be ready. I wanted to be able to present myself over the coming months as an able, responsible mother-to-be.

One of the first hurdles to overcome was the fact that I had always been messy. It was a family joke. Although much of my teenage years was spent cleaning toilets at the local campsite and turning down rooms in the local hotel for pocket money, I didn't give my own bedroom the same care and attention. My mother used to come into my room and find me lying asleep on the only clear space left on my bed, surrounded by clothes, cups and empty crisp packets among other things. However, instead of shouting, "Clean up your room, Deirdre, what a mess!" she would whip out her camera and begin snapping, all the while comparing my room to Tracey Emin's famous messy bed art piece, *My Bed*, which was famously displayed at the Tate Gallery and shortlisted for the Turner Prize... That's the kind of mother I wanted to be. But like all expectant mothers, I realised the responsibility that was coming my way, so I began to delve into some good books to try to teach myself how to declutter and manage my inherent messiness.

For any mothers-to-be, you really want to get yourself a copy of *The Life-Changing Magic of Tidying Up* by Marie Kondo (not to be mistaken for *The Life-Changing Magic of Not Giving a Fuck* by Sarah Knight – not so good for decluttering advice, but still a good read!). Marie Kondo teaches a technique through her book, which in simple terms asks you to only keep the things in your house that you really love and have a meaningful connection to. Hopefully your boyfriend, girlfriend, husband or wife will be one of these things, but perhaps your old clothes, books, shoes, photo frames might need to find a new home to create space for when the baby arrives. I also learned that it is a good idea to review what you have stored in the back of your cupboards and try to sell anything of value and make yourself some extra money!

Another area I needed to work on was managing money. I had never really considered, or appreciated, just how expensive babies could end up being if you're not well organised with your finances. After scanning the baby aisles in supermarkets and looking at the price of nappies, baby wipes and bottles, I began to wonder how on earth I was going to afford it all while also buying a new house. I was pretty miserable in my new job but I was just glad to be able to put some savings away. I didn't have any experience paying bills or managing money in the past, perhaps because I was never in a position of having enough of it! All I'd really had to worry about before was whether I had enough money for my next night out. An example of my frivolousness with cash is when I was flat broke at college and miraculously found a £20 note in a pocket of an old jacket. Instead of doing the responsible thing and thinking, *Fantastic! This will see me through the week! I can buy some food and go to the theatre*, I instead went out and bought some fishnet tights and a bottle of cheap cider. Needless to say, I'd been a pretty slim student with a lot to learn ahead of me. Now I had to really think about every penny I was earning and spending. Despite my lack of spending control in the past , I managed to learn a little about Excel spreadsheets in between doing some debt collecting in my job and this enabled me to capture my projected outgoings and income, which allowed us to see how we could begin to live within our means as a couple.

Compared to my progress with managing my finances, cooking was perhaps one area that would prove much trickier to fully turn around. Although I was the designated in-house breakfast chef at home when I was growing up and could make a mean fry-up, I didn't know much about the rules of a balanced diet, or what I should be eating to ensure that both the baby and I were getting enough of the right food. I needed to up my knowledge around nutrition – I couldn't rely on getting one of my five a day from the grapes in my Chardonnay any more.

My recipe for a meal went something like this:
- Open up the Domino's app.
- Add all the toppings, the sides and the dips.
- Place your order.
- After fifteen minutes, open the front door.
- Open the box and serve garnished with tomato sauce.

So to continue my journey of self-improvement, I decided to throw something together one cold March evening to impress Gary and give him a break from his cooking duties. After exchanging recipes with my mother, I settled for the Scottish classic, Cullen skink soup. I was out to impress and I really made an effort to nail the recipe. I wanted him to know that both he and the baby were in safe hands and that I could do better than just ordering a takeaway. I laid out candles on the kitchen table, which was set beautifully, and popped on our favourite playlist in the background to set the scene. The soup was on a slow simmer when Gary took his place at the dinner table.

"This smells delicious. Cullen skink is my favourite soup, did you know that?" he said, smiling over to me as he took his spoon and delved deep into the bowl of smoked haddock soup.

I waited in anticipation, hoping I'd seasoned it enough and that it wasn't too milky, or cold. And there it came, out of the bowl. With his first spoonful, he scooped up a small white dishcloth, just dangling at the end of his spoon. I had managed to cook the soup and the dishcloth together. This confirmed, very quickly, my position in the kitchen.

Luckily I had found someone who could throw together just about anything in the kitchen, and who agreed to teach me all about making delicious food. We spent time designing our food plans for the weeks ahead, to make sure that baby and I would be getting all the nutrients we needed to be healthy. I started to feel like time was against me. There were so many improvements I still felt I needed to make but I was making progress. I was embracing the unknown and becoming responsible for myself and our baby. I was growing up.

Judgement Day

It was judgement day. The day had arrived when I would find out whether I was going to be kept on in my job. I was hopeful that I would receive my forty-hour contract after my strong start at work. I was looking forward to breathing a sigh of relief and being able to put my money worries aside for a little while longer. This was the day I was to take the next steps to becoming a responsible citizen. The day I would get some added security for my new family. So I knew that I had to find the sexiest baggy dress out there to wear into the office, a dress that would allow me to look full of health and vitality, but not pregnant!

I patiently got through all my work and continued to tick off my targets until 2.30pm came around and it was my turn to be told whether or not I would be granted a full-time contract. Colleagues had been going in and out of the office all day, some returning to their desks with a smile on their face, others shuffling over quietly to clear out their lockers and head for the door. I began to realise how lucky the people heading for the door actually were – they were getting out of a desperate job. At the same time, I also realised how much I needed to be there for us all. After some reassuring conversations with my colleagues, I felt ready. The clock struck 2.30pm and it was my turn to face the music. I headed off into the manager's office carrying my brag file filled with my employee-of-the-week certificate and all the paperwork to back up everything I'd achieved to date. *No one has gone in with a BRAG file yet – I have this under control*, I thought. I felt ready to impress in my gorgeous new dress.

"How do you think you have done over the past five weeks, Sarah?" my boss asked. I ignored the fact he was calling me by my middle name.

"I feel I've settled in well. I've made some good friends and of course I have been employee of the week. You can see all my achievements here," I proudly stated.

"Very good, Sarah. Do you think there would be any issues with me continuing your contract?"

"Like what?"

"Well, it wouldn't be very fair of me to offer you a role when you'll be heading off soon, would it?"

He lifted his middle finger and pointed to my stomach. I began to crumble before him. I'd not been this shocked in four months.

Who told him? How does he know? What will I do? I remained speechless.

"Clear out your locker and leave the key on your desk, Sarah. Thanks."

"My name's Deirdre," I replied. As I left the room the full office turned to face me. I began to walk in what felt like slow motion to clear out my desk. Everyone dropped their heads after seeing my reaction and continued to work. I held back my tears with difficulty. I was so angry and embarrassed about the way I'd been treated. My pride was hurt too because I didn't expect to be let go. I felt I deserved to be kept on. As I began to clear out my desk, which was filled with 'good luck in your new role' cards, I also reached across to grab my mug that read *Girl Boss* – how ironic, I thought.

I headed home on the long commute from the office back to Gary. To his surprise I arrived home three hours earlier than normal. I just couldn't bring myself to call him to tell him what had happened. I needed to see him. To see his honest reaction when I told him that I couldn't even hold down a job.

"I got dismissed because I am pregnant. It was horrible," I said as he opened the front door and I broke down in tears.

Gary was furious about how I had been treated and wanted to take legal action against the bank that had fired me or at least make a formal complaint about the manager who had pointed to my baby bump before telling me I had to leave. However, he was more concerned with comforting me in that moment. He pulled me close to him and just said, "Oh, Deirdre, I am so sorry."

"I should be the one who's sorry," I said. "I'll try to get another job soon."

"No, you will not. It's nearly April and the baby will be here in August. I'll look after you both. You've been through enough. You need to relax and enjoy being pregnant. It's an amazing time for us both."

I spent the next few days calling around various employment law practices to see if I had some sort of a case, which of course I did, but I had very little energy to put up the fight. I felt discriminated against for being pregnant but I knew that with it being a zero-hour contract it would be a difficult case to win and in the end I just wanted to focus on having a happy pregnancy.

As the days began to roll by, I began to relax and get over the stress of losing my admittedly awful job. It was nice to let my belly relax and grow, and to feel all the sensations of pregnancy. I was coming up to sixteen weeks now and I was beginning to see some real changes in my body, the most obvious being a dark line that appeared at the bottom of my stomach, but my bump was still small and I was hopeful for a nice small (but very healthy) baby – one that wouldn't be too sore to push out!

Motherly Instincts

My inner gypsy was being tamed. I was leaving behind my carefree, self-indulgent existence and becoming a more responsible woman. I was learning to care for my body, for my growing baby and for the loving and meaningful relationship Gary and I had established. Life was speeding up and I was in the midst of the 'honeymoon period' of pregnancy.

I was making a real effort to stick to a healthier diet, switching from apple Pop Tarts to real apples, doing the opposite of Jesus and replacing wine with water and swapping our comfy couch for long walks in the fresh air. I was beginning to feel like a new person as my energy levels and health began to improve. It was nice to know what being healthy felt like. I'd missed this feeling! My new-found increase in energy levels was short-lived though, as getting a full night's sleep was starting to become a problem now that I needed to pee every few hours because of my developing baby pushing against my bladder. I guess that even my bladder was preparing me for the broken sleeps that lay ahead.

On some nights when my sleep was disturbed, I was able to have some late-night text exchanges with my eldest sister, Rachael, who had just left to go and start a new life in Vancouver. She was off to have the time of her life, a twenty-three-year-old living the *good life*. I was grateful for the time difference, as I enjoyed hearing her stories of adventure. It was an interesting juxtaposition with the type of adventure I had chosen to embark on, but we were both excited about the possibilities.

Hey sis – what you up to? I texted.

OK, so I met this really cool girl Alex and she's taking me to a rooftop pool party tonight. We've been drinking beer on a nudist beach today, so funny. Why are you up so late? she replied.

I had to go to the toilet again.

Have you got a bump yet?

Yes! I thought it would never come but each day I am waking up like WTF.

I still can't picture you with a bump, any other changes?

A few, but too embarrassing to mention.

Ha ha... I am going on a date tonight.

Already? You only just got there.

There's a lot of pretty people in Canada – so full of health!

OK, well let me know how it goes OK?

OK sis, night night X

We soon reached week twenty-one of pregnancy, another big milestone and another appointment. Gary also got some news of a new appointment – he had been applying for some jobs in the pharmaceutical industry. This is where he worked full-time before his DJ and music career took off. Although he made good money DJing and licensing some of the songs to TV adverts and computer games, he didn't feel it was a steady enough income to support a family. I don't think that it was his original plan to go back to work in the pharmaceutical industry but he really wanted to provide for us and he seemed very happy when he got the call to say he had been offered a new position. However, this new job meant that he had to travel to London to begin an eight-week training course. He came home every Friday though, so we still had our weekends together and my mum tried to support me as much as she could in between caring for Uncle Iain.

My mum arrived just before Gary had to leave for his first week in London, so that she could drive me to my second scan appointment.

"Should I find out the sex of the baby at the scan?" I shouted to Gary down the driveway as he got into his taxi to go to the airport.

"No, let's wait, we love surprises... don't we?" he shouted back at me, as he climbed into the backseat with a smile on his face.

It suddenly dawned on me how much I wanted to be able to drive by the time our baby was here. I thought about how it would give me a sense of control and independence. After all, I had already passed my theory test, so surely I could get my full licence in the next four months. I decided to add it to my ever-growing list of things to do.

It had been three years since my mother and I had been in a hospital situation together. The last time was after I collapsed at home due to appendicitis. It was a nerve-wracking two-hour ambulance drive to the nearest hospital in Inverness from Skye. I remember feeling worried that my appendix might burst – I knew that a burst appendix could be really serious – but at the same time, I was enjoying the buzz of the morphine and rapping along to Black Eyed Peas on the radio with my sunglasses on. I guess if it was going to burst, it was going to burst in style.

It felt really odd pulling up outside the Queen Mother's maternity ward in Glasgow with my mother beside me. It was such a surreal feeling that for a moment I felt like we could have been there to visit someone else. Usually my mother would have been accompanying her brother (my uncle) to his countless scan appointments or to meet with specialists. And here she was now, hoping to see a scan of the new life inside me.

As we walked inside I caught a glimpse of myself in the rotating glass doors. I realised how much I was still trying to conceal my pregnancy, wearing my red stiletto heels, tight jeans and tank top, like I wasn't going to let this baby get in the way of my fashion sense. Dressing up was something that I loved to do and I was really determined to win the fight against elasticated leggings and baggy tops with all the power I could muster. But I must admit, everything was beginning to feel a bit tight and uncomfortable.

"In you come, Deirdre," the midwife beckoned us in. "This is a very special day. You will hear your baby's heartbeat for the first time. Lie back here and we will take a look and have a listen."

I rolled my tight tank top up as far as my ever-growing breasts. Clasping my mum's hand tightly, I looked at her and imagined what it must be like for her to see her daughter in this situation. The little girl who used to stand on top of a chair to make her a cup of tea when she felt exhausted, the little girl who would pick bunches of flowers from the garden to make her perfume, the little girl who made her laugh, the little girl who always needed her. And there we were. Mother and daughter, listening to the heartbeat, loud and clear, of the first of a new generation. We just cried together. Tears of joy. Everything was overwhelmingly real now, a beating heart, so delicate and beautiful.

I was so excited by my mother's heartfelt reaction and I couldn't wait for her to see the scan which was coming next. There was far more to see now than at week twelve. The outline of a baby appeared. Tiny hands, feet, head, legs, arms and facial features. The heartbeat we heard belonged to the tiny baby growing inside of me and soon this baby would be mine to hold and take care of. There was a long silence as we both looked in awe at the slow movements of the baby as the sonographer clicked around the screen.

"I think you have a bicornuate womb," the midwife said, breaking the silence.

"Sorry what?" I asked in shock.

"You have a bicornuate womb, otherwise known as a heart-shaped uterus."

"Is the baby going to be OK?"

"Your baby is fine, but this can mean there may be a higher chance that you will need to have a caesarean section and the baby could arrive earlier than expected. It's nothing to worry about. This is just something you were born with. Pop off and let's weigh you. I think you should begin to increase your daily calorie intake slightly. Your baby's measurements are perfect, so this is just to make sure you're getting enough food," she added.

From the elation of seeing the outline of my baby and hearing its heartbeat, to the overwhelming panic of thinking something might be wrong, I realised my motherly instincts were beginning to kick in.

Mirror, Mirror on the Wall

Every item in my small wardrobe was beginning to feel tight and uncomfortable to wear. I was regrettably edging towards the day of wearing elasticated waistband leggings to support my bump, replacing tank tops with baggy tops and I was also in need of a larger-sized support bra. It was a bitter pill to swallow the day I had to reject my red stilettos but it was another exciting sign that I was getting closer to meeting our baby.

"My jeans don't come past my hips any more, Gary," I said, trying to manoeuvre my way into my favourite jeans.

"What about your leggings?" he questioned.

"They just about reach the bottom of my ass, but that's just not going to look good out in public. I need something with more of a stretch to it."

"OK, so let's go and buy you some nice maternity clothes?"

"*Nice* might be pushing it, but yes, I need something sensible, unfortunately."

"Where will we go?"

"I think Topshop has a maternity-wear section."

We drove into the city with me wearing a long jumper to cover my unzipped trousers. Topshop was a *big deal* for me growing up. It was the nearest clothes shop to my home in Skye, albeit a two-hour car journey away.

When we arrived at the shop I was immediately fixated by all the young women rummaging through the railings looking for size 6. This was the size I used to be and I felt slightly awkward in my new bigger body trying to find something that would fit. I remember feeling slightly envious of the other girls in the store with their slim figures. I still wanted to wear the tank tops, colourful dresses, skinny jeans, cropped T-shirts and sexy bikinis they were all off to try on, but it was time to size up and feel comfortable. I felt some eyes follow me around the store as I shopped. A few girls smiled at me noticing I was pregnant but I'm convinced that one or two had a sense of sorrow in their bright young eyes. I wondered if perhaps they felt fortunate that they weren't in my position. This was just another example of feeling like I was being judged by strangers. Part of it was due to my own anxiety about my ever-changing body.

"Do you think you'll be a medium in this?" Gary picked up a leggings-and-T-shirt bundle from the maternity section.

"A *medium*, me a *medium*, er, noooooo, I am a *small*," I said confidently.

"Oh, sorry, I just thought, er…"

"C'mon, pass me all the small stuff and I will go and try it on and show you. I haven't changed that much, Gary."

I entered the changing room with a bundle of maternity clothes, shaking my head in disbelief at the cheek of Gary. I began to manoeuvre myself out of my jeans and carefully slipped myself into what felt like my new identity.

"Can you get my boyfriend?" I peeked my head out of the changing room and asked the retail assistant a few moments later.

"Everything OK in there?" Gary asked.

"Just take all of this and swap it for a medium or large."

"Oh, OK. Are you OK?"

I couldn't answer. I stared deep into the bright unflattering mirrors. Everything was bigger. My cotton bra and pants looked like something I would see hanging off my grandmother's clothes line. My thighs were beginning to touch at the top. My face resembled a hamster with a week's supply of food stored in its cheeks. My boobs were beginning to burst out of my comfort bra, I had a ballooning belly and I could see noticeable stretch marks across my stomach. It was a glorious sight for all the wrong reasons. Change wasn't just coming. It was already here.

Walk of Life

It was coming up to week twenty-three of my pregnancy, and my body was continuing to astonish me. I was increasingly aware of the sensation of a living baby inside me. Now that I could feel this beautiful new life growing inside of me I felt a sense of wonder that really helped alleviate some of the anxiety that I was experiencing about my changing appearance. I'd managed to get away with staying out of the public eye for a while, partly because I spent a lot of time in Glasgow trying to plan for the future, including keeping up with my few scheduled driving lessons and planning for our new home, and partly because I was a little bit unsure of myself and hadn't fully adjusted to my new identity as mother-to-be – this new identity, after all, was a long way away from my previous alter egos Debbie Ferguson and Diane Rutherford. However, one of my older sisters, Eilidh, was turning twenty-one and her birthday celebrations were to coincide with a fundraiser for my uncle's hospice. It was time to face my first public appearance back home in Skye, bump and all.

During my successful trip to Topshop, the one which made me feel even more pregnant, I managed to fall for a beautiful black dress, which the bump and I could squeeze into. After applying spray tan, fake eyelashes and make-up, I just about resembled the old me. I remember having a real glow about me on that night and I was beginning to appreciate the miracle of pregnancy and was starting to see the beauty in my changing body and developing bump.

I'd met a lot of pregnant ladies at parties in the past. You would usually see them surrounded by people congratulating them, touching their bump, hugging them and making a real fuss over them. As I thought about this, I became nervous about what people's reactions might be when they saw me. Was everyone going to have the same type of positive reaction like the one I was hoping for? Or would people stare and judge me?

Skye is a very small community where everyone knows everyone's business and showing up to a party nineteen and pregnant definitely drew out a few interesting reactions and looks, but only from the people who didn't really know me or my situation. They hadn't even met Gary, and didn't have any knowledge of how in love we were.

I made my way around the room, confidently selling raffle tickets, calmly taking compliments, and enjoying the feelings of being in control and letting my hair down. I began to feel a little bit more confident in myself and really appreciated all the kind words and compliments I was receiving from people I knew in the community. Despite all the worry, once again it wasn't anywhere near as uncomfortable as I thought it might be. Besides, the spotlight really wasn't on me that night. It was on my uncle. He was a true light in a lot of people's lives on the island. The event that we had organised with him raised thousands of pounds to support the hospice that was caring for him and others in a similar position.

I watched my sister as she danced around the room, having fun on the eve of her twenty-first birthday. She was surrounded by all her friends and family and looked to be in her element. As I observed her, I wondered what my twenty-first birthday would be like. Would I look as free as her or would I be stuck at home changing nappies? Would I ever look that good again, or would I let myself go? Would I be surrounded by friends or would I be surrounded by potties?

I remember the moment when the DJ played 'The Walk of Life' by Dire Straits. This was a special request for my sister who was famously born in Raigmore Hospital in Inverness while this song played on the radio. Being pregnant really makes you think about life, love and family and as I got swept up in the fun of the moment I remember contemplating how we were beginning to walk our own paths in life and how we often can't plan for the things that destiny has in store for us.

The following morning after the party I was the first one up out of bed – things were definitely changing! As I walked through my childhood home, stepping over the mess and empty beer bottles from last night's after party, I realised I had forgotten what a hangover felt like. I made my way into the birthday girl's bedroom.

"How does it feel to be twenty-one?" I bent over Eilidh's bed and asked her.

"Horrific. Hangovers suck! Please make me French toast and bacon. You know you're the best person at making breakfasts," she begged.

"You're just saying that so I'll make it."

"Well, you need to get some practice in so you can make the baby some decent food, right?"

"Again, this is blackmail – but OK, obviously I will make you breakfast!"

I realised in a split-second that I was already playing the role of mum. The mother whose automatic job was to wake up and make sure her children were fed and watered. I cooked with great pride.

"Kids, that's your breakfast ready! Hurry up before it gets cold!"

Bodies began to appear from all around the house. One by one each of my family and friends began to stumble into the kitchen like extras from the *Walking Dead*. The involuntary moans and groans they were all making was enough to remind me what it was like to have a hangover and I actually felt really grateful that drink was off the menu for me. I was getting used to being the one who felt good the morning after any nights out or family parties. As they all sat down around the dining table, I recalled the moment a few months before when I stood in the same position announcing my pregnancy. Now I was standing in front of them all with my developing bump, flipping rashers of bacon onto their plates and feeding Millie secretly under the table. I realised in that moment that I was beginning to enjoy my new-found maternal and motherly instincts. Maybe I was cut out for the role of being a mum after all.

"Thank you, sis, I told you you were the best at making breakfast," my sister spoke rudely through a mouthful of bacon.

"She sure is, she is becoming quite the chef," Gary added, thankfully forgetting all about the Cullen skink.

"How did it feel last night, with everyone from school there and even some of your teachers?" my sister asked.

"I felt pretty good actually. I've spent so many months worrying about what people think of me, when all I should really be worried about is becoming a good mum and being the best girlfriend I can be."

"Well, you're certainly going in the right direction with this fry-up, Deirdre!" Gary joked as the table broke down in laughter.

After breakfast I decided to take a walk outside to get some fresh air and gather my thoughts. As I sat down on the shore outside my home, I realised how different my surroundings looked and felt now. The shore that used to be my playground where I searched for crabs and razorfish seemed much smaller now; the house seemed smaller. I was beginning to see everything in a new light. I don't think I had ever fully appreciated my childhood until that exact moment. I stared across the glittering sea to the Isle of Raasay, watching the seals sunbathing on rocks only yards in front of me. I took deep inhalations of the clean sea air, listening to the sounds of chattering birds in the background. I was beginning to understand it all now. I was beginning to see why my parents had worked so hard to give us a life here. I had a new-found appreciation for everything that my family had done for me and I became aware of my own sense of yearning to provide the same type of stability for my own family.

Filtered World

Nowadays almost nothing you see online and in magazines is a true reflection of reality. People always post the best pictures of themselves and you can pretty much guarantee that those pictures have some type of filter applied to help everything look perfect and unblemished. When you see pictures of pregnant women in magazines, they have usually been airbrushed within an inch of their life. With their perfect skin, stretch-mark-free bellies, salon hair and teeth that could make you blind if you stare too long, you know instinctively that nobody in the real world could ever actually look THAT perfect when pregnant. However, despite this knowledge, it can seem impossible not to compare yourself to these images of perfection while you sit there with your baggy pregnancy pants, one leg draped over a maternity pillow and a face fit for a no-make-up selfie. With all the empowerment that choosing to become a mother brings, there are still going to be times when your self-esteem feels a little bit jaded as you fight the inevitable tiredness, body blues and ever-increasing urge to be the perfect mother-to-be.

I knew I had to find some tools to manage my wavering self-esteem, especially living in the modern world, where social media makes it hard not to compare yourself to other people from your big toe to your earlobe. I was still getting to know social media, how it worked, how many times a day I should be posting pictures of my food and what the best lighting was for a selfie. I was also quickly learning that you get a lot more likes if you have a baby or a pug in your pictures. It really is a very shallow world but it's part of our culture now and although I'm not a huge fan of it, it did help me keep in touch with the friends and family I was seeing less and less of as the months went by. It also gave me a bit of a laugh when I inevitably ended up comparing my situation to all of my friends' when they posted exciting updates detailing their adventures. It went a bit like this:

We just booked our round-the-world ticket!

I'm like – *I think I have another stretch mark forming. FML.*

OMG, I just got into drama school.

I'm like – *Eh, I think I might need to swap these size medium leggings for large ones, Gary.*

I'm moving to New York in the summer!

I'm like – *Is* Jeremy Kyle *on repeat today because I need to go to my scan appointment.*

Who's coming out tonight?

I'm like – *Think I'm going to treat myself to a bag of Doritos and some Mad Men on the TV.*

Anyone up for coming to T in the Park this year?

I'm like – *Can someone get me a cold glass of milk? I've got indigestion.*

No matter how hard you try, you will inevitably compare yourself in some way to others, whether it be online, in magazines or in life. In some ways, it's part of human nature, so you need to forgive yourself for it. My uncle decided to teach me a technique that he had picked up at a self-help conference that he had attended to help him cope with his cancer. He had learned a lot but decided to share a simple affirmation with me that he thought would help. He explained that your mind generally believes what you tell it. If you tell yourself you're not good enough, then you won't feel good enough; if you focus on your flaws, then you'll ignore all the good things about yourself. He told me that he now began each morning with a mantra spoken into the mirror, and encouraged me to do the same, every single morning from now on. I didn't particularly enjoy spending time staring at myself in the mirror, but now I found myself standing each morning really studying myself. Looking beyond the surface. Looking at the real me. Just me and the mirror. My freckles, spots, the gap between my teeth, the green eyes, the trashy dyed-blonde hair, the pale complexion, the dimpled chin, the shape of my nose, the scar from my bike accident on my forehead, my baby fringe, my short eyelashes.

I began my mantra: "I'm beautiful, I'm beautiful, I'm beautiful."

I told myself out loud that I was beautiful, over and over again, to try to look a little deeper, to try to look at myself in a whole new light. This was how I now started all my days and if at times I felt anxious or scared I came back to my mantra until it calmed me. Perhaps I was just going along with it for him, but it helped and I continued to build on my confidence and appreciation for all the work my body was doing for my baby. Ironically there are sometimes negative things said about positive thinking, but I found that it really worked despite my initial scepticism. If one mantra doesn't work for you, you can change it to suit yourself, just as long as it's something really positive.

"I'm beautiful, I'm beautiful, I'm beautiful." You should try it. *I dare you.*

Out with the Old, In with the New

You could say pregnancy is the gift that keeps on giving. Every time you think you've got the hang of it, there are always more surprises waiting around the corner. By week twenty-six, I was glowing on the outside but weird things were still happening to my body on the inside. I had now accepted that the ever-expanding size of, well, *everything*, was just part of the magic of pregnancy, but now my body was throwing in some extra discharge and thrush to keep me on my toes. After googling my symptoms I concluded that what I was experiencing was thrush. At that point I should have stopped googling and phoned my midwife, but I was interested to know what the possible safe treatments might be. One bizarre treatment I found told me I should soak a tampon in natural yoghurt and stick that in my vagina every two hours. I was horrified, so I called my midwife for advice and she reassured me that thrush was a natural symptom of pregnancy and there were many ways to clear it up without sticking natural yoghurt up my nether regions. There must have been a lot of cervical fluid production going on up there, I could feel it! So I was glad that it was considered normal and nothing to be concerned about. However, I've never looked at a pot of natural yoghurt in the same way again since!

Every day there was yet another slight change.

Oh my goodness, my nipples, they are getting bigger every day!

Are those lumps on my nipples?

Eh, I actually think they might be changing colour. Is this normal?

Oh no, there's more stretch marks, on my inner thighs? WHY?

What's happening to my belly button? Why is it beginning to stick out like that?

I need to go out and buy another bra size, this one is going to burst.

I only shaved my armpits yesterday, why am I getting so hairy?

Why do my feet look chubby? My feet?

On the plus side, Gary thought I looked gorgeous. He was endlessly fascinated with my bump, not to mention my expanding breasts, and he always told me that I looked radiant and sexy while pregnant. Maybe he was just being nice but now that I think back, our sex life was still pretty good during my pregnancy when I wasn't feeling too self-conscious. This is yet more proof that a lot of the worry and concern I was feeling about my appearance was mostly unnecessary and admittedly a little silly at times.

As my pregnancy progressed and we began to prepare ourselves and our lives for our future son or daughter's arrival, it felt like we were studying for some kind of project or university course together. A course that we had both picked on a subject that we knew absolutely nothing about! We both felt we had so much to learn about babies and parenthood. We just hoped that after all the preparation and study we would pass the test and become fully qualified parents. We learned that baby may now be able to hear us, and were encouraged by the midwife to start talking to him or her, so that it would feel comforted by the voices of its future mum and dad. I was grateful for the knowledge that the baby was only beginning to hear now. If it had been able to hear me any earlier, I'm almost certain that its first thought after being delivered would have been something along the lines of *Oh, shit, help me!* or *I want to go back in, you're not ready to be my mum!*

On the weekends and evenings that Gary was home from his training in London, we started a bit of a tradition of reading chapters out loud from our favourite books, hoping that our little baby would enjoy the stories and the sound of our voices. From *The Alchemist* to *The Way of the Peaceful Warrior*, we relished the fact that baby could hear us and that one day we would be able to teach this baby how to read.

There seemed to be more calmness now; the dust was settling, just in time for the phone call to let us know that we could now collect the keys to our new home. We were spending almost all of our free time in places like IKEA, baby stores and B&Q. We were leading a completely different life to the spontaneous carefree romance we had been caught up in only months before. We still managed to keep our Friday movie nights locked in and anyway, I was really starting to enjoy shopping for all the things we needed for baby and our new home. I guess you could say I was in the nesting phase of pregnancy. This is another interesting phenomenon where pregnant women get an almost uncontrollable urge and overwhelming desire to clean and organise their homes. I can't say that I felt that strongly about cleaning and organising but I was definitely enjoying this phase a lot more than I thought I would.

Finally the weekend arrived when we pulled up outside the estate agent's to collect the keys for our new home. We felt ready to take one further step towards being responsible parents. Holding the envelope, I reminisced about how the last anticipated envelope I held had told me I was heading to New York, and now this one was telling me that my life was going to be settling down for a while. It was a sharp contrast but I distinctly remember having the same feeling of optimism and excitement about the future. Who would've thought that that outgoing party girl would become so excited about settling down. Everything was starting to come together.

The Second Trimester:

A summary of what's happening to you and your baby & the things I wish I had known

Welcome to the 'honeymoon period' also known as the 'second trimester' – I can hear you: *Why is she saying honeymoon period? Now that I am entering week fourteen is everything just going to be blissfully smooth?* Er, no. The phrase *honeymoon period* comes from the knowledge that the days ahead should bring more energy, your sex drive may return and hopefully the nausea and fatigue will subside as you enter this new phase of your pregnancy feeling a bit more like, dare I say it, the old you!

What Cool Things Are Going to Happen This Trimester?

- You will be offered a screening scan which is primarily to check the growth and development of the baby – all major organs are screened for structural abnormalities such as heart conditions. If the sonography finds any abnormalities such as cleft lip and palate, etc, you will be told and further discussions will take place. Although this scan can also determine what sex your baby is, which is super cool (if you want to know), it is best to be aware of all the possible outcomes of this important screening scan.
- You'll see your baby on the screen again – prepare to be AMAZED!
- You will start to feel movement inside.
- Your baby will begin to recognise Mum and Dad's voice.
- Your antenatal classes will be booked.

While you go through this phase of having some unexpected energy, begin to have a think of everything you want to do before baby gets here. You should still be feeling pretty mobile and the bump shouldn't be getting in the way of you getting things done. Suck every moment of this time up, it doesn't last long!

- Considering a baby shower? Now is the time to get planning!
- What about planning a romantic babymoon together before the baby arrives? It will never be just the two of you again!
- Start to discuss baby names – you will be amazed at how long this process can take and you only have around fifteen weeks to decide!
- Have a look at local childcare facilities in your area – if you know you are going back to work childcare spaces can fill up very quickly so get your baby's name down on the waiting list!
- Start to have a look into breastfeeding, the benefits it will give to your baby and how to best prepare for it.
- Begin to shop around for the essentials you'll need when baby gets here – don't get carried away!
- Have you got any pets? Now would be a good time to arrange some care for them during the time you are expecting.
- Make sure you have confirmed your maternity / paternity arrangements with your workplace.

Your Body

You'll be beginning to put on extra weight as your bump develops throughout the trimester. I remember from my screening scan that I had been told to make sure I was eating enough; I had a tiny frame, and not a huge appetite generally but it did push me in the direction to maybe eat a little more and embrace my changing shape. Although I thought my bump was small during the second trimester I now know that even if I did have a small baby it wouldn't really mean I would have an easier birth; births are all so different, and the actual ease of the birth will mostly be dependent on many different factors, not the size. Your baby in the second trimester begins to swallow fluid known as 'amniotic fluid' which contains nutrients, hormones and antibodies to fight infection. As they practise swallowing and digesting, it's good to keep yourself on the right track with all the nutrients you are supplying your body with.

When it comes to what you are fuelling your bump with, everything you eat or drink while pregnant reaches your baby and has an influence on their overall health.

- Vitamin D and calcium will help your baby develop healthy bones and teeth.
- Omega 3 (found in nuts and fish) will improve the baby's brain and eye development.
- Folic acid will help support spine development.
- Protein is good for their muscles, organs and bone tissue.

I really began to see change during this period – here are a few common changes to expect.

You'll get a free boob job

Yes, the tingly sore breasts will be replaced with expanding breasts as they prepare for feeding – you will gradually be going up in size but keep supporting them! I went up three cup sizes in the space of six months – you may begin to develop stretch marks as your skin tries to keep up with the fast-paced growth.

This is all happening for a reason, and the reason is you are going to be able to feed your baby! Pretty cool, huh?

Backache

As you begin to put weight on more quickly over this trimester, your growing bump will begin to place extra pressure on your lower back. Make sure you stay active throughout the day, you're not picking up anything too heavy and that you're sitting comfortably and supported at work.

Discharge

Yes, it's not going away with pregnancy and it's so normal to see a thin, milky vaginal discharge throughout pregnancy. If you think it might be turning into an infection do advise your doctor. Signs of infections include itchy, offensive smelling and/or discoloured discharge.

Swelling

Your body is producing around 50 per cent more blood and body fluids to meet the needs of your developing baby, which in turn can cause areas of the body to swell, including your hands, face, legs, ankles and feet.

Hair growth

You may feel yourself getting a bit hairy in places (and not just on your head!) but this is *natural* and is down to those pregnancy hormones again! Hopefully you will feel like *'You're worth it'*, but if you are sprouting hair out of your chin don't panic – it's only temporary. Once your baby comes out so will your extra hair!

Linea nigra

Don't worry I'm not going all Latin on you. A dark line may be appearing, running from your belly button down to the pubic area, during this trimester. It's your pregnancy hormones that are responsible for this darker colour. It's actually always been there, you just can't see it – and it will fade once your baby is out.

Acne

Did you miss having spots in your teenage years? Although you can expect to glow during this trimester, you may also begin to develop some breakouts. Again, this is down to hormones, this time called androgens, and should clear up. It's just part of the process.

What's that smell?

An unusual, yet common side to pregnancy is that your sense of smell may change, or even more odd, your smell might change. It might be as simple as the smell of, let's say, Peperami makes your mouth water but pasta might make you feel queasy.

Stretch marks

It would appear that no amount of Bio-Oil or trips to Lush for creams keeps the stretch marks from forming. Stretch marks appear when your body begins to grow faster than your skin can keep up with. As you continue to put on weight and baby grows this can put a lot of pressure on your growing skin, and stretch marks may not just appear on your bump, but also other areas like your bum, thighs, breasts and upper arms. I wish I could tell you there is a miracle cure, but there is no treatment that can prevent this from happening, but you *can* control how you feel about stretch marks.

- You're not alone – more than half of women develop stretch marks during pregnancy.
- Rapid weight gain can bring stretch marks on so stay within your suggested calorie intake.
- Stay calm – your stretch marks, although they may seem bright, will over time fade to thin white lines which no one will notice.
- Keep hydrated by drinking plenty of water and keep stocked up on vitamin C – it probably won't prevent stretch marks, but it will keep your skin feeling nourished and moisturised!
- *Embrace them* – stretch marks will be your last concern once baby arrives and I think they are just another mark of how awesome us women are!

Heartburn and indigestion

Due to a hormone called progesterone this can bring on heartburn and indigestion. (The hormones are at it again!) Heartburn is very common in pregnancy and there are a few ways to help relieve the symptoms. I found it often came on worse at night-time, so always have your remedies in easy reach.

- Cold glasses of milk – the dairy or non-dairy kind (my magical cure).
- Don't overindulge; eat smaller meals throughout the day.
- Foods to think about avoiding – spicy food/tomato/ citrus fruits/coffee or greasy food! Burny!
- Try to avoid doing eating and drinking at the same time, as this can bring on acid reflux.

If none of these remedies seem to work, speak to your local pharmacist about others that can help prevent it.

Oral health

Another important part of your body to look after during pregnancy is your teeth! Due to all the hormone changes you become at higher risk of developing gum disease, which in turn could be harmful to the baby. We all cringe at the thought of going to the dentist, but I wouldn't be telling you if it wasn't important, so get the fluoride toothpaste out and start brushing!

- Keep your teeth as clean as you can and get into flossing!
- Tell your dentist you're pregnant and advise them of any medication or prenatal vitamins you are taking.
- Visit your dentist during each trimester so they can clean your teeth and examine your gums.

UTIs and thrush

Yes, this book just keeps getting better, doesn't it? I'm a long-term sufferer of urinary tract infections (UTIs) and it's something that is common during this phase of pregnancy. As your hormones change, they can slow down the flow of urine, causing the bladder to not empty fully as the growing uterus pushes against it. Although it is common, you want to get in touch with your doctor if you experience any of the following:

- Burning sensation when urinating.
- Having to urinate even more than is normal during pregnancy.
- If you have blood in your urine.
- If your urine has a strong smell.

Don't worry, it's not all that bad – oh no, wait a minute, I haven't told you about *thrush* yet, have I? White, milky discharge is another normal symptom during pregnancy. It's not harmful, but if it becomes thick, white, begins to resemble cottage cheese and is causing itchy sensations in your vaginal area, it's most likely to be thrush and you really want to do something about it!

- Thrush doesn't harm your unborn baby.
- Speak to your doctor or pharmacist about your thrush and how to treat it.

Tips on how to try to avoid it:

- Wear cotton underwear and change daily (obviously).
- Make sure you wash your underwear in a hot wash.
- Change out of swimsuits/exercise clothing as soon as you can.
- If you are using pads, change them regularly.
- Avoid using products that might irritate your skin and 'that area'.

Getting to sleep

Sleep is something all us pregnant women crave, yet it can sometimes be hard to get to sleep. Although anxieties at this point may be lessening, your baby is now growing quickly, which means your uterus will be pushing against your bladder. This will leave you needing to pee a lot and can interrupt you during the night. You may also find yourself tossing and turning as you try to get yourself comfortable; and you may also begin to experience some crazy dreams as your sleep cycle becomes more interrupted. I spent many nights dreaming that my waters were breaking! Who knew sleeping could be so difficult!

- Try not to drink too much before you plan to fall asleep.

- Make sure you are comfortable – pregnancy pillows are a great way to give your bump support and keep you in a good position!
- Exercising during the day and being out in the fresh air can help you sleep better at night.
- Your brain is busy, so take time to relax before going to bed – practising some meditation before sleep can really help.
- Have a warm bubble bath to help you unwind.
- If your partner is complaining because you have all of a sudden become a snoring machine, tell him to buy some earplugs.

Exercise

Did someone say *extra fries*? Exercise might not be your thing, but burning calories by dancing on tables in a nightclub is no longer an option – and you want to keep moving. Pregnancy actually got me back into thinking about the great outdoors again and I loved getting out walking in the fresh air. If you are used to exercising regularly, there are many exercises you can still enjoy while being pregnant; and if you are new to it, it's the perfect time to give it a shot.

For those who are new to it, it is recommended to follow a gradual progression of exercise and having an achievable target of 10 minute bouts per day and building up to a total of the recommended 150 minutes per week of moderate-intensity exercise. Running, jogging, racquet sports and strenuous strength training may be less suitable for those just starting exercise and if you have any queries about what you should and shouldn't partake in do speak to your midwife about what would be suitable for you.

Exercise will not only be a form of escapism for your busy

head, it will begin to make you feel more energised and look healthier. Look out for local pregnancy fitness classes in your area. Some good exercise options for you include:

- Swimming
- Brisk walks
- Indoor cycling
- Gentle aerobics
- Yoga or Pilates

Toilet habits

Remember how I mentioned it's a good idea to introduce some fibre into your diet? Well, constipation is caused by the hormone progesterone, which relaxes and smoothes the muscles throughout the body, including the digestive tract. This means that food passes through your intestines more slowly; later in pregnancy, the pressure of your growing uterus on your rectum can slow the pooping process right down. You may also begin to have some embarrassing flatulence issues; again this is another symptom down to the increase in progesterone – but don't worry it should pass (if you'll pardon the pun). Here are some tips to help:

- High-fibre foods – wholegrain cereals and breads, brown rice, fresh fruits and vegetables.
- Make sure you are drinking plenty of fluids – even mix up your water intake with some fruit juices to help get things moving!
- If you gotta go, you gotta go – don't put off going to the bathroom – *for anyone.*
- Exercise can relieve constipation.

Cyberspace

During my pregnancy, I had a love–hate relationship with the Internet. It answered a lot of questions – at least, I think it did – but there is so much information out there that you want to make sure you are sticking to good content! I remember the day I googled images of childbirth was the day it really sunk in that this human was actually going to get out of me somehow. But I got sucked in quickly and before I knew it I had terrified myself by reading horror stories on forums telling me how awful pregnancy is, which in turn made me feel awful! And with the horror comes the counter-gloating, which brings in all the insecurities that build up inside you! STOP comparing yourself to others. There is plenty to think about without the added anxiety of worrying if you are going to be as good a mother as all the mummy bloggers on Instagram.

Friendships

It's great to make some friends outside of the Internet too, you know. There are some real people out there who, like you, are reading this book wishing they had someone to talk to, going through all their own worries. If you are the first in your family or groups of friends to have a baby, it might be worth looking around and recruiting some new ones. Although your old friends will still love you, they will be too busy partying, shopping and dating to worry if you have a working breast pump at home. Patience is a key with friendships, old and new; your relationship with them will be different now, and all they'll want is to spend time with old you, which, somewhere down the transition into motherhood, you may lose.

- Be open to your friends about how you are feeling.
- Make time for your friends, even after your baby

comes along.

- Check local mum meet-ups, coffee mornings or pregnancy talks – you just don't know who you are going to bump into – and if you don't have any in your area maybe set one up. Mothers have loads to talk about!
- You will be coming up to attending antenatal classes where you will meet other women in a similar position; don't be shy to reach out.
- Speak to your midwife about other mothers your age at the same stage as you – maybe she can make an introduction.
- Introduce yourself to people at your antenatal classes; they are in the same position as you. Many mothers meet life-long friends in these classes.

Your Baby's Growth in the Second Trimester

By the end of the second trimester, you will have around a two-pound baby in your tummy! Your baby is still developing rapidly and this month your body will begin to take a new shape as your bump gradually becomes larger. Prepare to fall in love at your ultrasounds. If your pregnancy didn't seem real up until now, well, now you'll feel it. (Literally!) So go to your appointments with some tissues.

Weeks 13–16

What if I told you your baby may be able to suck its thumb? Cute or what! Your baby is now about the size of a large avocado! All their limbs and joints are fully formed and they will be getting stronger every day. Their nervous system is also making connections to all their muscles so the baby may begin to move a little more. They may also be preparing for the school playground as they begin to grip and play with their umbilical cord!

Weeks 17–20

Your baby is growing very quickly! All their organs are now formed and his/her lungs are beginning to function. Hair, eyelashes and eyebrows are beginning to grow. As well as its eyesight, your baby will also begin to hear sounds outside the body, so careful with your language! If you are noticing more movement, it's just your baby exercising their developing muscles!

Weeks 21–24

You might begin to feel your baby hiccup! Your baby will also be developing its own sleeping pattern, which you will soon get used to. Your baby's skin and brain are developing rapidly at this stage. If you are having a baby girl, guess what? Your baby girl will develop eggs in her ovaries during this month. If you're having a baby boy, now is when his testicles descend into his scrotum. How amazing is that? We were born to mate! Although still relatively small, your baby is now almost fully formed and is taking the shape of a real human!

As you begin to feel your baby move around it is always good to keep a close eye on movement and if you have concerns over your baby's movements go get it checked out.

Shopping List for YOU During the Second Trimester

- Panty liners – yes, just when you thought you were getting away with it for nine months – they are essential if you are experiencing any leaks/discharge.
- Comfy, stretchy clothing from top to toe!
- Sleeping masks to assist with sleeping.
- Pregnancy books to help you gain some insight or ease

your worries!
- Moisturiser for your belly.

Shopping List for Your BABY During the Second Trimester

While you have some energy, start to get ready for baby coming! It won't be long now!

- A chair that supports you when feeding your child in the night.
- Baby clothes – don't go mad though, you still don't know the size of your baby!
- Changing table – you will need a safe, clean place to change your baby.
- Moses basket for your baby to sleep in for its first few months.
- Baby bathtub.
- Baby bedding – a few changes of sheets and a good mattress.
- Nursery accessories – but don't go crazy! They really don't remember how pretty their nursery was!
- A small teddy – this will be its first teddy, which they'll never want to part with!

PS

You are now entering your final trimester. There is still a lot of growing to do, but you will be getting more organised, more educated and more at one with your pregnancy and looking forward to the arrival of your baby. It's normal to still feel an array of emotions. No one has ever said, 'I had the most blissful pregnancy,' unless they were in denial. As you move forward into days of more change, keep reminding yourself of how important you are, how your body is able to produce a human being and how, regardless of all your anxieties, you will be a great mother.

Reflections

Change wasn't alien to me. I'd changed a lot over the years leading up to my pregnancy. Body changes, life changes, mood changes. I was quite comfortable with change. I think it's one of those things you just need to be open to. I changed even at school on a daily basis, depending on what crowd I was hanging out with. I changed to make myself look prettier when I was around Gary. I forced myself to change and grow that first night in Glasgow when I felt insecure. I changed my name so people would think I was older. I changed the way I dressed so I could work in an office. It's amazing how much we all can adapt and change, sometimes without even really realising it.

I knew change was something I was going to have to deal with throughout pregnancy. The truth is, I was actually a little bit bored of the party-girl me. My pregnancy came along at the right time, even if it didn't make sense to others. I was ready to change into someone more responsible, someone who could morph into a motherly role. It was a change and a challenge in itself, but I was ready to test my willpower, face all my fears head-on and accept the hand I had been dealt.

I didn't dwell much on my body image growing up. Perhaps I'm grateful that Mark Zuckerberg is only six years older than me and he was still in halls of residence typing in codes to his computer before launching social media platforms when I was at school, because growing up is tough enough without following Victoria's Secret models on Instagram. I grew up in an era when I didn't have to compare myself to anyone.

I was lucky.

I was a size-six, peach-bum, perky-breasted nineteen-year-old. (I know, total bitch, right?) I'd never really looked at myself and appreciated all the bits and bobs that made me *me*.

I knew that changes in my body were maybe going to be the most challenging changes of them all, but there comes a point where you need to see the beauty in it all. It's a choice, how you view yourself. Positive reinforcement is key. Instead of dwelling on the parts that are changing that you can't control, spend your energy focusing on how your body can do all this in the first place, how it knows what to do to grow a baby! Something definitely happened to me as I progressed through my pregnancy. Maybe it was my mantra, but there was a fear within me that was beginning to fade when I looked in the mirror at myself. We've been having babies for millennia. Angelina Jolie's had twins and she's bloody gorgeous!

It's so easy to compare ourselves to these celebrities. I have been guilty of comparing myself to so many people I don't even know, women from all corners of the globe who appear to be better mothers than me online. But one day I just stopped. I had to learn not to compare and instead to learn from them. Perhaps my developing relationship with the Internet filled a bit of a gap when loneliness crept in. Being online was and still is at times a distraction. You can connect to new friends around the world who have similar interests to you and get an insight into the lives of other mothers out there. I know 'friends' is a bit of an overstatement: they don't even follow me back. But as you settle into your own journey some of your friendships may be tested as you find yourself with less in common with them. One of the Internet's purposes is to bring people together and I guess I was gaining new online friends in a really bizarre, pathetically uncool way.

After all, they are just people like you and me, wanting to reach out, wanting to be part of something – just like I wanted to be part of something when I was pregnant. They're just people like you and me who get that warm fuzzy feeling when someone likes their post. Just another character in the story. And just because my character didn't always have a tidy house like theirs, or a fancy car like theirs, or a bookcase like theirs, or a bowl full of hand-picked organic fruits from their local farmhouse, didn't mean my character was any less special. I am my own character, you are yours.

Pregnancy did teach me something about friendship: you really need to value and cherish the ones that you have. Your true friends will stand out above the rest. You'll know them, and you'll love them more now than you ever thought possible. And even if there are times that the loneliness creeps in because you don't feel like anyone around you really knows what you're going through at each stage of your pregnancy, talk to them. They'll help and they'll WANT to help and listen to you. And I mean the real-life human friends, not the ones that you follow on Instagram. The ones that will take you out for a hot chocolate and marshmallows at midnight, the ones that will answer your call when you discover the discharge for the first time, the ones that will lift you up when you start to see your body changing. That's what friends are for.

And if you're feeling so lonely and afraid to talk that you don't know where to turn or who to speak to, speak to your midwife. There's never a stupid feeling or question when it comes to pregnancy, and you're hearing that from the one that asked her midwife if she should stick natural yoghurt in her vagina.

Because of the love bubble I was in with Gary I didn't really reach out to people my age that were going through the same thing. Instead I ended up treating pregnancy like picking a really weird subject at school. Throughout my second trimester, through to the end, I did endless research on the Internet and in books, so I was constantly learning. I actually think I may have read more books about pregnancy than I ever did for my geography exam (don't tell my parents). For every book that made me feel inadequate (one, written by Myleene Klass called *My Bump and Me*, only managed to make me feel extremely ugly as I flicked through it and mostly focused on how different to her I looked in my pregnant state… There's that old comparing thing again – DON'T DO IT!), there were also some really great resources that I picked up and read, which filled me with promise and hope and filled in the gaps in my knowledge about pregnancy and motherhood – especially the Pinter & Martin books.

Something was definitely changing within me as I developed through my pregnancy. I became softer. More loving. More grateful. The selfish eighteen-year-old party girl was leaving me, and I knew I was becoming a better person. I look back and realise that although at times I was hard on myself, I needn't have been, because I was doing pretty well – just like you'll be doing.

The responsibility of being in control of someone's life is really life-changing.

PART 3

The Third Trimester

Lucky to Have You

I decided to take the train from Glasgow to meet my mother for a mother-and-daughter weekend in Inverness. We timed it with my uncle's visit to the Highland Hospice so that we could spend time with him. Sometimes the hospice, which supported my mother from a distance, needed to have my uncle stay over in order to tweak the complex medication he was on and to give my mother respite. I really missed my uncle so I was glad that I would get to see him. I remember thinking that this would be the last weekend my mother and I would spend together before I too became a mother. We hadn't been able to spend as much time together as we'd have liked during my pregnancy, as my mum had thrown herself into caring for her sick brother, nursing him in his own home and temporarily moving in to give full attention to his needs. She knew from the moment we got the news that his cancer was terminal that he would become her focus.

He was an impossibly likeable guy. He was funny, kind-hearted and had lived life to the full. Friends gravitated towards him. We, his nieces and nephews, became the centre of his universe. He took a huge interest in all of us and my pregnancy elated him. He wanted so badly to be here for the baby's birth.

When mum and I arrived at the hospice, his eyes lit up when he saw me and my growing bump.

"How long now, Deirdre? When am I going to get to meet the wee one, or big one by the looks of things?" he asked, looking more frail than he did three weeks before at his fundraiser.

"It's due in around nine weeks, Uncle Iain, and you better be back home by then and have the champagne at the ready to wet the baby's head!" I responded.

"You bet your bottom dollar I will be. I'm as excited to see this baby as if it was my own grandchild! I kind of regret not having had children of my own, but you guys have become my surrogate family anyway!"

My uncle had been married for a few short years but it hadn't worked out. He'd had other relationships with various women since his marriage broke up; he certainly didn't have any trouble in that department. But the right person just never seemed to come along and he never remarried. He used to tell this hilarious story of a singles' holiday he'd signed up for on the Greek island of Symi.

On the plane from Glasgow to Rhodes, he'd had a few gin and tonics. When he arrived in Rhodes he made his way to the harbour to board the two-hour ferry to Symi. The boat was full to capacity, and he relaxed on the deck, basking in the sunshine, trying to work out which passengers might be on the same holiday as him. He decided it was time for a refreshment so went down to the bar and ordered an ice-cold beer. A fairly plump, wrinkled woman of about sixty-five sidled up to him. He would have been about fifty at the time.

"Hi, where are you from?" he said.

"I'm from Plymouth," she replied.

"Are you meeting friends on Symi?" he asked.

"No, I'm going on a singles' holiday!"

He wondered what he was letting himself in for, but being the perfect gentleman, he bought her a beer and they enjoyed the rest of the ferry trip together.

The boat approached Symi, and on first impressions, it

looked like an idyllic island. They were met off the boat and taken to their accommodation, which offered stunning views over Symi harbour. When my uncle had settled in, he got to know the other singles over a few welcome drinks. The wine was flowing and everyone was getting on famously. He took a sip of wine and suddenly there was a stinging sensation in his mouth. He had been bitten by a wasp! Soon his mouth began to balloon up. This was not a great start to his chances of finding love on the trip! After dinner, and with the help of free-flowing wine, he managed to forget that his lip was the size of a whale's. The group partied on, hitting the bars, until before he knew it, it was 5.30am. His first night ended in a haze of new encounters; memories of individual conversations were not going to last long!

Later the next day, he spotted the other singles having a beer in a local bar. He decided to join them. Everyone was getting on really well, when all of a sudden the woman he had met on the ferry appeared.

"What are you doing here? You said last night you were going to meet me at my apartment." She ranted on for a few more minutes in full view of the whole bar, which was extremely busy.

There was a deathly hush as she picked up his pint of beer and threw it over his head. Not satisfied with this, she picked up his friend's beer and poured that over him as well! Next, she slapped him round the face. By that time my uncle was beginning to feel slightly annoyed. He felt he had two options at that point. Either add to the scene by retaliating, or walk away. He chose the latter!

The next day, the woman from Plymouth appeared at his apartment full of apologies for her behaviour. He told her the best thing she could do was leave him alone for the rest of the holiday but this didn't happen. He was stalked for the rest of the week, being peeped at from narrow doorways and alleyways; she was always just a stone's throw away, making him jump out of his skin. The holiday had become a nightmare!

A few nights later, his singles group decided to go for a few beers to their favourite local, which was situated high up on the hillside overlooking Symi harbour. The pub was buzzing and everyone was having a great time. All of a sudden the bar door burst open.

"Hello, I am Mr Klein! My yacht has just sunk in the harbour and I have about £50,000 of insurance money here to spend!"

Everyone was speechless.

"I want to buy everyone here a bottle of wine to celebrate!" he told them.

True to his word he bought the whole bar a bottle of wine each! The party was in full swing. My uncle was sitting right beside Mr Klein. Behind them there was a small room where about twenty people were enjoying their night.

"When I was in Russia, the people all drink like this," Mr Klein told him.

At that point, Mr Klein downed his shot of vodka, and threw his glass over his head, hitting one of the guys in the other room on the head. It burst open and his face was covered in blood. All hell broke loose! My uncle decided that fighting wasn't the best way forward and stepped in to successfully calm everyone down. Mr Klein made his way to the bar, where the manageress told him to get out.

"I am not moving from here," he said.

At that point, the barmaid took a huge baton from behind her and went to start hitting him with it. My uncle was standing right beside him and took the full brunt of this attack. Mr Klein decided enough was enough and left the premises.

This was a typical story that left me in tears of laughter! And this from a hospice bedside, when you would at least have expected a more sombre conversation. His pain management was going well. He had been pain free for about ten hours the day before, which he told me was the first time in ten months he had felt so good. His morphine dose had been raised so he was sleeping more. My other memory of that visit was his gratefulness for the high calibre of care he received from the doctors and nurses. He thought they were just superb, nothing was too much trouble, and they were all up for a good laugh, which meant he was in his element. I loved seeing him in such good form, as my mum and I left for lunch.

We sat down at the table.

"I really wish I was allowed to eat shellfish," I said. "I really miss it."

"You can have shellfish if you want. A small amount of shellfish, as long as it's thoroughly cooked won't do you any harm."

"Can I take your order?" the waiter asked.

"Could we have the scallop starter – it needs to be well done, my daughter is pregnant – two risottos and a large a bottle of water, please?"

I looked across the table at her and felt a real sense of love and appreciation for her. Despite all of the energy it took for her to care for my uncle, she was still being a mum and looking after me.

"How did you think your uncle looked?" my mum asked.

"I'm surprised about how positive he is. He seems determined to see this baby. It's given me a real boost to know how much this baby means to him."

"I'm finding it hard to reconcile the fact that I'm going to be a granny and lose a brother in a small space of time. I find it hard that I can't be down south offering you more support and keeping you company. But at least you come home regularly to see Iain and me, so for me that's a huge bonus. Is there anything that you're worried about?"

"I sometimes feel like a rabbit caught in the headlights. I don't know what I've let myself in for."

"These nine months are like a magical mystery tour, aren't they? No book can really get across everything that you feel, and all the changes that happen to your body in rapid succession. Motherhood will change you in more ways than you can imagine, but you will adapt, that's for sure!"

"I just can't fully imagine myself in that role yet. You know, breastfeeding and all that. Of course, I'll give it a go! I just can't imagine myself doing it."

"It should come naturally to you. It's very instinctual. For some, including myself, it can be a struggle. There are quite a lot of factors that come into play for breastfeeding to work well for mother and baby. Things like baby latching on, a stress-free environment, the ability to relax. And I'm sure other components too but I'm no expert!"

"It doesn't sound like it's going to be much fun, to be honest!"

"Maybe not fun at first but it's a journey like any other. It's a bumpy road to travel but the rewards are immense! I can't honestly get across how truly beautiful an experience it is to love and care for your own child! And look at you – you have youth on your side!"

"I'm not sure if that's a positive or a negative."

"Horses for courses really. You will be blessed with more energy for the job at hand than I had, being a new mum at the ripe old age of thirty! I was actually considered an older mum back then! Interesting how perceptions change. It wasn't that unusual for woman to have children around your age in the previous generation."

"But you had five! Were you some kind of masochist? I guess I'm still trying to figure out who I am and what my purpose in life is. I don't want this baby coming into the world and growing up with a confused mother."

"As soon as you hold the baby in your arms, you will look at life differently, trust me. It will change your perspective on absolutely everything. You'll realise it's not all about you any more. To be a parent you have to become somewhat selfless and it's actually very empowering. It sounds counterintuitive but you will understand when the time comes. Also, having a baby isn't going to change who you are. You are just going to become more than you are and more than you thought you could be."

"I'm just worried I'm going to lose myself. All my dreams seem like they will be impossible to achieve once I become a mum."

"Oh, come on, Deirdre! You are nineteen years old. You have your whole life ahead of you. Most parents go on to pursue their careers and dreams. The only thing stopping you from doing that is YOU, not your children."

"But so many don't. I don't even have a job, Mum. I literally don't know if I have what it takes to be a good mum."

"You have a great partner. Not everyone has that, so you should be grateful that you have each other for support. You will be amazed at what you're capable of when you become a mother. I knew nothing about parenthood either before I had my first child. No one does. But somehow the world keeps revolving and people keep having babies. You have to have some faith in your instincts and when it comes to your dreams, you just need to remember to make time for yourself when you can. What you want might change when you become a parent and it might take longer to achieve what you're aiming for, but you'll get there if you are determined to succeed."

I thought about my uncle lying in bed in the hospice across the river from where we were eating lunch. I wondered what it must feel like to know that there isn't much time left. I felt very sad for my uncle whose light was going to be extinguished too soon and I also felt guilty for worrying about the prospect of bringing a new life into this world. The contrast was very stark in that moment. Life and death. The beginning. The end. The cycle of life. It was heartbreakingly bittersweet. In the days that followed, my uncle sadly began to deteriorate. He was transported back to Skye to spend his final weeks or months at home, where he wanted to be, surrounded by his family. I decided to spend some more time in Skye to help nurse my uncle. I just really hoped and prayed he would still be here when his new niece or nephew arrived within the next few months.

Back to School

I was nearing week thirty and it was time to attend my first antenatal class back in Glasgow. My uncle was in a comfortable position and implored me to go, hoping the education would help me feel more confident and reassured about what to expect during labour and beyond.

Gary and I arrived at the Queen Mother's Hospital in Glasgow feeling a slight sense of nervousness about the class and what it would be like. As we were taken in, I scanned the other couples as we searched for two empty seats together. It was clear that we were the youngest couple in the room by quite a number of years. We began to learn the ins and outs of what was going on inside my body and how to best prepare for labour, learning new words like 'pelvic floor' and 'colostrum'. We discussed positions that may be helpful, most of which looked like something only flexible people could achieve. I began to wonder if I should have taken up yoga as I'd heard it helps prepare you for childbirth. *I'm ruined,* I thought. *My youthful vagina is going to be destroyed in a matter of weeks and for what? A lifetime of responsibility*. I wondered if Gary would even be able to look at my vagina in the same way again after he had witnessed it eject a seven to eight pound baby. As women we're all aware that having a baby is billed as being one of the most beautiful and wondrous things you can do on this earth, but if we're all being honest with ourselves, it also sort of resembles a scene out of a horror film!

When I got comfortable in my seat, we were told that there would be a short presentation on the screen. As I looked up at the screen, I was transported back to a conversation I had had with a fellow actor on the Meisner training course as we walked through Times Square.

We had stopped for a moment to look at our surroundings, taking in the mesmerising images from the hundreds of bright, colourful screens surrounding us. The screens were filled with the most famous actors, models, musicians and presenters in the world. It felt like they were sort of looking down at us as we wandered through New York's most famous square.

"Your face is going to be up on those screens one day," he said.

"I doubt that very much, but thanks, that's very sweet of you," I replied.

"I'm telling you, you will be up there. I knew as soon as you walked into class there was something special about you. I can't put my finger on it but you have that magic thing that people talk about. I think you could be very famous one day."

I shrugged my shoulders and smiled as we continued walking the blocks to class.

The thought of becoming a master at the craft of acting and preparing for a difficult role in a film or play actually seemed like an achievable goal now when compared to the preparation needed to master the role of becoming a mother. A role which required me to be responsible for another human being, for their whole life long. I knew it was going to take a lot of work but I also knew, like any difficult role, I would get there with it.

I snapped out of my daydream when the phrase 'birthing plan' was mentioned. A *birthing plan*? I thought you just went to hospital to have a baby. I didn't realise that people choose to have babies in their *homes on purpose* with limited pain relief!

Wow. I had really learned something at this class: we women are unstoppable! I began to put my birthing plan together in my head:

- *9am – I will wake up after a restful night's sleep on my due date with a few cramps and head to the hospital.*
- *10am – I will be taken up to my room in the maternity ward and be given some pain relief to take the edge off, so I don't feel anything.*
- *10.30am – After a few relaxing breaths and bounces on a yoga ball I will lie back and Gary will hold my legs in the air and I will gently push.*
- *11am – A beautifully wrapped, healthy baby boy or girl will be placed in my arms.*
- *11.30am – A hair-and-make-up artist will arrive so I can look as good as Kate Middleton did when she had her baby.*
- *12.00pm – I'll tuck into some delicious food, make some phone calls and text friends to let them know I've survived while my baby sleeps angelically by my side.*

"I will see you all in two weeks' time and remember to get your hospital bag prepared in case your baby comes early," said the midwife, bringing me back to reality.

The class had passed very quickly, just like everything in pregnancy. Labour and having a baby requires some real grit, determination and skill. There's lots to think about and do while in labour. A lot of it happens automatically and with the help of the doctors and nurses at your bedside, but there is still a lot of effort involved for the mothers and the partners too, if they are present. In that short hour, I learned a lot but most significantly, I learned a new appreciation for what my mum went through when she had me.

Before I reached the car I began to put a list together of things to follow up on. I began my pelvic floor exercises (basically tightening your vagina to strengthen your muscles) to build up a strong pelvic floor. I turned to my shell-shocked other half as we got into his car.

"I've started doing my pelvic floor exercises," I stated proudly.

"That's good," he replied.

"It's actually quite pleasurable, and no one knows I am doing it."

"Well, at least you can now say you do one form of exercise," he joked.

"Very funny! Do you think I should take up yoga?"

"I think you are actually really flexible and strong."

"I did actually do ballet for three weeks when I was younger. I just want to be as prepared as I can for labour."

"Do you think you learned anything from that class?" he asked.

"Yes, it's that that no vagina is equipped for that. I mean, can you actually believe that something weighing maybe six to ten pounds can come out of a woman like that? It's at times like this I wish I had a penis!"

"Are you still doing your exercises?"

"Yes, and genuinely enjoying it."

"Good. Now let's go home and a pack a bag."

Have You Got a Fast Car?

I returned to Skye to help support my family with my uncle, and also to take what I thought was another massive step in my preparation for motherhood. It was an important piece of the jigsaw for me. I had finally booked a driving test!

I saw the driving examiner gawp as I left my dad's car and waddled towards his silver Skoda at the starting point for the test. I was struggling to keep composure as I heaved my heavily pregnant body into the driving seat. He regained his composure and joined me in the car. He obviously hadn't got the memo that he was going to be driven by a hormonal, tired, heavily pregnant young mum-to-be that day.

"Hello, I'm Deirdre, and I'm not fat, there is a baby in here," I said, hoping for a laugh.

"OK, can you please pull out of this lay-by and continue down this road," he responded in monotone. He obviously didn't appreciate my joke.

I made sure the instructor knew how much discomfort I was in when I got into his car. I thought it may actually win me some sympathy points for my assessment but he seemed immune to my charms! It really was a massive effort to go through with my test so close to my due date. The effort involved wasn't just because I was pregnant; it was also because I hadn't had any practice driving on this stretch of road before the test. All my driving practice had been in Glasgow, so the night before I sat down and thought about all the possible difficulties I may encounter on Skye and prepared a map of possible routes. The hazards I may face included wandering sheep, single track roads and hitchhikers – all very different from the city driving I'd been doing in Glasgow.

The examiner took a deep breath and I began to drive nervously, dictating my prepared monologue as the test progressed, "Seven weeks today I am due. I'm so glad that there was space for me to sit my driving test before the baby comes. I mean, can you imagine how bad it would be if I couldn't even drive when my baby arrives? How would I be able to get to the shops when I run out of nappies or wipes? Or go anywhere for that matter! It would cost a fortune in taxis. There's just no way I'm going to have time to sit another test after the baby comes, I'll be so busy. I really hope I do OK."

There was a long silence until he spoke, "Can you do a three-point turn up here?"

Suddenly memories came flooding back of me practising a three-point turn in my driveway at the age of twelve. I'd asked my uncle to stand at the end of the driveway and watch me work my magic. The only magic I created that day was crashing into the back and front doors of my mother's new car, which had only arrived the previous night. I took a deep breath and tried to erase the memory of my younger self losing control of the steering wheel. This time around, I managed to perform the three-point turn immaculately.

The quickest hour of my life passed and my dream of being able to drive rested entirely on the results. The examiner turned to me and looked me in the eye and said: "Well, Deirdre, you have passed!"

I was so elated that I actually wanted to kiss the assessor but I held my composure and graciously shook his hand and thanked him for his time. After saying goodbye, I spent the next minute awkwardly trying to manoeuvre my way out of the car. It was embarrassing but I eventually managed to escape with a little help from the man who just gave me a pass on my driving test. I couldn't wait to share the news with my dad who was coming to pick me up.

"I passed," I screamed, quietly, trying not to frighten the baby.

"I had a feeling you might pass! That map you made last night – that was pure genius. You'd visualised any possible hazards in advance. Well done!" my father said.

"Thank you!" I replied, smugly.

"Well, at least you have another thing ticked off your list!"

I asked for permission to borrow a car to drive to Glasgow that day. I wanted to surprise Gary by turning up in the driveway. I'd spent many of my formative years being envious of older siblings and friends passing their driving tests before me, picking up friends and boyfriends, cruising and doing doughnut spins in the car park.

But now it was my turn. I sat there in the car I'd borrowed from my parents with a 200-mile journey ahead of me to reach the city. Just me, baby and my mix tape. It was the first time I'd driven alone and it was exhilarating. I rolled down the windows, turned my mix tape up full blast, looked in awe at the beautiful landscape as I drove through the beautiful Scottish Highlands. I sang my little heart out as I drove and relished in the freedom I felt. I was in the driver's seat now.

Cravings and Nesting

I'd spent many of my pregnant months looking forward to the day that I would experience my 'craving' for something unexpected. "Have you had any cravings yet?" I was often asked. I was in the depths of my final trimester, but still nothing, aside from a slight craving for milk and salt. Most mothers I spoke to about cravings had some strange stories to tell me about what they craved to chew on, some of the highlights being coal and grapefruit, and the least fortunate one being dog biscuits. I was hoping for something nicer to get my teeth into, like strawberry ice cream or jars of peanut butter.

It was around 10pm after one of Gary and my date nights at the cinema that my first real craving struck! We had just begun the twenty-minute dark drive home from the cinema when a sense of panic and urgency took hold of me. I instructed Gary to pull over at the nearest petrol station with great haste.

"Do you need to pee?" he asked.

"Surprisingly no, I just need to pop in for something."

I got out of the car and power-walked to the store with a sense of great purpose. Gary really must have thought that something was wrong or that I actually was about to pee my pants and just didn't want to tell him.

"Do you have any more of these?" I asked the man behind the counter.

"No, that's the last box," he answered, with a concerned look.

"Right, I'll just take what you have left then."

The man was speechless. He took my cash and his eyes followed me with interest as I left the shop and rushed towards Gary's car with the biggest smile on my face. I closed the car door and sat down next to Gary holding around twelve red hot and spicy Peperamis. He also stared at me with concerned eyes like the cashier had moments before in the shop. I frantically opened my first stick of salty, spicy meaty goodness and took my first frenzied bite. It was a glorious feeling. I had satisfied my craving. This was it. This was what I needed in my life. A dirty red hot and spicy Peperami! It was pure heaven. Gary put the windows down to get rid of the smell and laughed at the bizarre sight he was witnessing. It definitely wasn't sexy, but I didn't care. I was also very glad that Gary didn't want a bite, because I wasn't up for sharing!

Our renovation project was starting to come together and our house was starting to resemble the type of home that I would want to bring up a child in and one that we could start to build our family's future in. I could now see a future with the three of us settled in our cosy little home. The list of improvements needing doing was getting smaller and as the workmen began to move out, the decorators moved in to complete the finishing touches. Even though we were definitely getting there, we continued to tour homewares stores and baby shops for little things that we still needed. Who would have known that such small beings would need so much stuff? IKEA was beginning to feel like a second home at this point. The only thing that got me through those last trips there was the prize of a hot dog and an ice-cream cone at the payment counter. I really was craving some pretty bad junk food but I was still conscious of my overall nutrition and health so I allowed myself to indulge from time to time.

The more our house began to feel like a home the more I didn't want to leave it. I heard an old wives' tale that it can be a sign that baby is almost ready to arrive when the nesting phase gets more intense. I tried to control my overriding desire to finish organising my new home, but sometimes the urge was too strong.

Gary caught a glimpse of me late one night when he accompanied me on one of my cleaning missions. He was downstairs and I was in the bathroom. I decided that I wanted to scrub the grout in between the tiles so I stripped off my clothes to avoid getting dirty and got to work. As I leaned over the bath, belly balancing over the side, with nothing but yellow marigolds, a pregnancy bra and an ill-fitting pair of tight leopard-print knickers on to preserve my modesty, I realised that this would be a bad moment for Gary to walk in and see me. But as I scrubbed the tiles, I heard a voice coming from behind me.

"You are one of the sexiest cleaners I've ever cast my eye on," my Gary gasped.

"Are you trying to tell me you've had the pleasure of witnessing something like this before, Gary?"

We spent the next five minutes laughing at how ridiculous I looked.

As much as I felt I was having to do a lot of growing up in a short space of time to prepare myself for becoming a mother, it was all starting to make sense and I was now feeling more content and less overwhelmed with fear and anxiety about the future. I had the car, the home, the man and a baby on the way. The house was almost finished, I had learned to look after myself better and I could now cook a decent meal. I felt like I had really come a long way over the last eight months. Maybe I was becoming a responsible adult a little faster than

I had planned but I was evolving and getting my shit together – it felt empowering.

Where Is My Mind?

I was becoming aware that I was beginning to lose it a little from time to time. So-called 'baby brain' is a *real* problem. I spent many hours looking for my mobile phone only to find it in the fridge hours later. I pretended to be a dog and barked at my boyfriend when he arrived home from work one day, and sometimes I completely forgot what I was saying mid-sentence, leaving many people confused, and worried, for the baby's future. Although I often found these little episodes amusing, I didn't want to appear unhinged to the people I was coming into contact with. I decided that I was going to let myself off lightly when I made a fool of myself as it was just another part of being pregnant. Like I said before – it's the gift that keeps on giving! You just need to go easy on yourself when you inevitably make mistakes or have an attack of 'baby brain'.

The baby was very lively in the morning now and morning baths began to look like something out of *Alien*. There was a lot of movement going on and sometimes you could just make out the shape of an arm, a leg, or a head as baby moved itself around. I also thought I couldn't possibly get any bigger at this late stage but each day I'd find it harder and harder to fasten my dressing gown and there was no chance of getting into my leopard-print pants now to do the cleaning, much to Gary's disappointment.

Gary and I continued going to antenatal classes, even though they sometimes seemed intent on making me more nervous than ever. One week we arrived to find a crying baby of the human variety, as opposed to the doll variety, being presented to the group. The baby girl was only two days old and the pretty woman who was holding her looked extremely tired and worn out like she'd been through an exhausting ordeal. I could hear my own heart thumping as I imagined myself in the delivery room pushing and screaming expletives as Gary and the midwives looked on with concern. It's amazing what your mind can make you feel when you let it run wild. Once I had snapped out of my little panic fantasy I could see the proud look on the new mother's face and although she looked tired, you could feel the happiness and joy she was exuding as she allowed us to interact with her perfect little newborn.

Wow!

I had never seen a baby so young before. She had tiny feet and tiny toes. A little scrunched up face like a bud waiting to unfold. A hint of a smile pushed her cute little lips up the sides of her delicate face. For someone who wasn't really a big fan of babies in the past, I was taken aback by how much I wanted to hold and touch her. I remember thinking that lady and her baby was going to be me soon. I would soon be holding my own child in my arms. I started to think about the miracle of how we as women are able to create, carry, deliver and raise these tiny little human beings. It really is a wondrous thing. I almost, dare I say it, in that moment, felt ready.

Being pregnant over the summer months is manageable in Scotland, because the weather during July and August can sometimes be more like a winter's day. I was glad not to have to make too much effort to look *hot*. The end was in sight and I was actually getting to the point where I was looking forward to giving birth as everything went from uncomfortable to batshit crazy in the final month. My once average-sized tits now looked like cow-sized udders, I was using my bump as my own personal dining table, pimples were beginning to appear on my tired-looking face and Gary had affectionately renamed me 'Penguin' because of my ever-worsening waddle.

I was ready to lock the doors and stay out of sight until it was time to go to the delivery room, so you can imagine my dismay when we were invited to a garden party at my good friend Pixie's house. It was no ordinary garden party either, she was turning twenty-one and she had gone to the effort of setting up a gazebo. She wasn't going to take no for an answer and I felt obliged to make the extra effort to attend. On the day of the party, as I tried my best to get out of my faithful elastic (now large-sized) leggings and into the summer dress I intended to wear, I caught a glimpse of myself in the mirror and felt like I was getting dressed up for a Hallowe'en party, not a garden party. Nothing was working. No dress could tame the enormous bump now, no bra size could tame the massive breasts, no comfy shoes could tame the swollen feet and no amount of spicy Peperamis could tame my appetite.

There was no point trying to hide it any more. I had no choice but to let it all hang out. I waddled my way, slowly, downstairs to see Gary. I had become a walking, talking, living caricature of a very heavily pregnant woman.

"Can I get you anything?" he asked, forgetting to comment on how hideous I looked in my dress.

"Can you get me anything? *Can* you get me anything? Ha ha ha! Yes, Gary, can you *get me* someone to carry and have this baby for me? You could maybe even get me a hairdresser and make-up artist. Could you please also get me an electric chair to take me up and down the stairs? What about something to stop my humongous breasts leaking everywhere? While you're at it, can you confirm that I still actually have feet because I haven't seen them in weeks? Can you start lifting me in and out of the bathtub and maybe stop looking at me like I am an accident waiting to happen?"

Wow – I wasn't really angry with Gary but my emotions and hormones were running the show now and I clearly needed to let off steam. I just wanted the floor to swallow me whole at that point. I was so embarrassed by my outburst. I was fed up, heavy, sore and leaky. I was still freaking out a little about going into labour but the discomfort I was feeling started to make giving birth seem like it might actually be a relief!

Instead of taking any offence from my nonsensical outburst, Gary held me and just said not to worry. He suggested that I climb out of my summer dress and get back into my faithful leggings. He told me that he would push the couches together so that I could watch chick flicks all day while he looked after me. He was right, I needed to relax. I had got myself into a state. He told me that I would need to arrive fashionably late to the garden party, and that the dress actually looked really pretty on me given the circumstances. Now I was crying because I remembered he really loves me and I could tell that he was genuinely sorry I felt like this. As I got myself comfy on the couch, it wasn't long before I was crying again although this time it was over an advert on TV for life insurance. I really was an emotional car crash that day.

Ah, the third trimester. It's a lot of fun!

All You Need Is Love

Gary and I decided to spend some more time in Skye as my uncle's illness began to reach its final stages. The hospice had told us that his life expectancy could be days or weeks and that he was nearing the end. It was really difficult to see him now. He had lost so much weight and looked so frail and fragile. We had only seen him a few weeks earlier when he still had a sense of humour and the ability to laugh, talk and engage with everyone. Now he was drifting in and out of consciousness and didn't have much energy to speak. I remember being glad that I had been able to travel to Skye to spend time with him throughout his illness. I was also very grateful for the last outing I had with him just weeks earlier. He was on good form that day and was very chatty. Gary and I took him for a long walk in his wheelchair along the coast. We had some really deep and meaningful conversations about what's really important for a life well lived and what may lay ahead for us all in the great beyond after death.

My uncle was very much a family man. He told me to keep the people I love close and to cherish every minute I got to spend with them. You never have enough time to say and do everything you want to with the people you love in life, no matter how long you live, he told me. You really have to remember that time is finite and that each moment is a gift. He said I should try to remember this each day if I can. He also said that if I have any regrets about not making the most of the time I had, I should be kind to myself, as life is way too important to be taken seriously all the time. Alongside some of the nuggets of wisdom he was sharing with Gary and me, he also wanted to talk about what might happen after death. This was a very difficult thing to talk about at first but Uncle Iain wanted to discuss it and hear our thoughts. He also pushed us to be honest about it. As we talked, we covered a lot of big topics and questions such as whether there was a heaven or an afterlife. Did we all come from a singularity and if so, are we all one? Can you even have life without death as they both need to exist to make either a reality? If we were all created by the same energy when the big bang happened, then do we ever actually die or do we just eventually take a different form because energy can't be created or destroyed, because according to the laws of physics, it can only change forms? I have to admit that I was getting a little confused once physics came into the equation but Gary and my uncle were really getting into all the different theories and possibilities that lay beyond. I was so glad that Gary had got to know my uncle. They really liked each other and got on so well. I was really going to miss him when he went and so was Gary.

As much as I didn't want this visit to end due to my uncle's deteriorating health, Gary and I were committed (on Iain's earlier orders) to attend our final antenatal class in Glasgow. Before I left the house, he had taken my hand in his and placed it on my bump. We spent time in this position as the baby moved and kicked. As he felt the baby move he whispered how lucky I was to have met such a nice guy and how lucky this baby was to have us both. I turned to him and whispered, "I'm lucky to have you." I leaned over the bed he was lying in and gave him the biggest, longest kiss with my bright red lipstick. I left the room holding back tears, telling him that I would be back in two days and that it wouldn't be long now until the baby arrived.

We arrived at the class just in time to see all the couples being told to get down on all fours. The classes were very educational, albeit slightly cringeworthy at times, due to the various positions they made us practise. I learned some breathing exercises that were meant to help during labour and Gary learned some skills for keeping me calm and encouraged. We were given lots of props, such as yoga mats and giant birthing balls, and taught lots of exercises and techniques to help with labour, delivery and beyond. I remember spending most of the class in denial. I couldn't believe this was my last class. The baby's arrival was only weeks away now. Where had all the time gone? As my final antenatal class drew to a close I remember expecting some kind of fanfare or at least a farewell slice of cake, but all we got was a pleasant handshake and good luck wishes as all the parents-to-be were sent on their way. As Gary and I left hand in hand, I noticed my phone light up in my handbag with a missed call. A feeling of panic went right through me as I knew instinctively why the missed call was there.

"He's gone."

"I'm so sorry, Mum."

"He was at peace, surrounded by his family in his home, just what he wanted."

It was the saddest moment of my whole life. My sweet uncle was gone and I was heartbroken. I wept for hours, unable to grasp the fact that I would never touch him, have a conversation with him, listen to his funny stories, take him for walks along the coastal road in his wheelchair or drive with the rooftop down in his midlife-crisis convertible listening to the Beatles blasting while the rain poured in on us. Gary was also devastated, but he did his best to comfort me and remind me that although he was gone in the physical sense, he would still live on in our hearts and memories and we would be able to tell his future niece or nephew all about the type of person he was and pass on all his stories and wisdom to the next generation and beyond. I took comfort in this thought and it reminded me of my uncle's theory that although our bodies die, our energy lives on forever. Although he had gone in the physical sense, I could still feel his love and the presence of his energy all around me. I felt so lucky to have known him and although he would never get to meet my baby in person, he got to share most of my pregnancy with me and for that I was very grateful as I knew it made him very happy.

I was nearing full term after my uncle's funeral in Skye, so I had to leave my grief-stricken family for Glasgow to spend my final days as a free girl and await the first signs of labour. On one of the warmer summer days, I managed to squeeze the baby and me into a little black dress, then added my oversized sunglasses and a pair of Chelsea boots. I hit the West End to wander around the art galleries and visit my favourite coffee shops, taking advantage of the peace and quiet before my baby arrived.

My bump was certainly catching the eyes of many passers-by, who looked at me curiously as I made my way around Kelvingrove Art Gallery. I could see some onlookers whisper to each other and stare, a few concerned nods from elderly people, and a few 'oh dear' looks from what looked like new students exploring their city. Although I was beginning to feel good from within, I couldn't help but feel slightly awkward about some of the looks I was getting.

I decided to take myself down to the gallery cafe for a bowl of soup. The most beautiful young waitress came along with my bill at the end.

"Can I just say something to you?" she asked through her

warm smile.

"Yes, of course," I replied curiously.

"You are the most beautiful pregnant lady I have ever seen, you look really cool."

"Oh my goodness, thank you!"

"You're going to be a seriously cool mum."

I left her a £5 tip and waddled quickly to the toilet as tears began to form under my dark sunglasses. I felt amazing. She thought I was a lady and she called me beautiful. It was so kind of this lovely stranger to pay me such a perfect compliment just when I needed it. The kindness of strangers is truly a wonderful thing.

Labour Day

There are a lot of horror stories out there about childbirth, and if I'm honest, having been in slight shock for half my pregnancy, I hadn't had much time to dwell on how this baby was actually getting out. My labour story sadly isn't as straightforward as it appeared in my head when putting my own birthing plan together.

It all began at 2.45am on Sunday 16 August 2009. I was woken up in Gary's parents' house by a strange cramping feeling, just like they had spoken about in class. I was alone in bed, waiting for Gary to return after his Saturday night DJ set in Glasgow. I knew this was it. I just lay there on top of the bed, stopwatch in hand, counting the space between contractions. There was no going back; this was happening and my massive bump was going to turn into a crying, pooping, hungry child very soon. I heard the front door close downstairs and chuckled to myself at Gary's attempt to sneak quietly up the stairs. Little did he know that his pregnant girlfriend was wide awake upstairs and already in the starting phase of labour.

"It's happening," I said as he peeked into the bedroom.

"How many minutes?" he replied, quietly trying not to wake his parents.

"Around five minutes apart."

We tiptoed quietly down to the living room, staring at each other in a stunned silence only broken by momentary fits of nervous laughter. It was now around 3.40am. We woke up

Gary's parents and we all gathered around the kitchen table. Gary's mum sorted everyone out with a cup of tea and some toast to keep us all going. I knew it was still early in the process, and that this was actually the early labour stage they spoke of in class, so I took the opportunity to give myself a final pamper before the inevitable trip to the labour ward.

I had always been concerned about how awful I was going to look during childbirth, so a well-thought-out plan was put into place to give me as much dignity as possible. One of my prebirth plans to get a full body wax was scuppered when I became so afraid the baby might pop out if I screamed too hard in pain. At the very least now, I had some time to shave my legs. Shaving is extremely difficult with a giant watermelon belly in the way, but you can find ways to get around that. I then painted my nails, pulled on my brand-new sexy knee-high socks and slipped on my new night-dress. I stared at myself in the mirror and began to laugh at my attempt to make myself look somewhat pretty, as I was most certainly going to end up looking pretty awful in a few hours anyway. I just wanted to make a little bit of effort to make myself feel just a little less self-conscious, and being organised enough to get the basics done really helped.

Not my usual Saturday night look, I thought to myself!

My contractions started at around 2.45am and it was now 4 in the afternoon. The contractions were closer together at this point so we got in the car and drove towards the hospital. They were also becoming more painful so I used some of my breathing exercises on the way to the hospital to settle my nerves and take my focus off the pain. We arrived at the hospital and I got my examination – which I cannot stress enough *is not the same as the exams you sit at school*. It involved a glove and a couple of fingers which were unceremoniously pushed up my vajayjay. Don't get me wrong: they were very gentle with me, but this was not what I was expecting. I was subsequently turned away, because I was only 2cm dilated and therefore not ready to be taken up to the maternity floor. I was now seventeen hours into my labour but I was being asked to leave the hospital and rest for a few more hours until I was at least 4cm dilated. I couldn't believe I was being sent home this long into labour. I was already starting to feel very tired and I worried that when it eventually came time to push I'd be too tired to do anything.

We decided to drive to the flat I used to share with my sister, who still lived there, as it was located near to the hospital. Gary went for a nap but there was no way I could sleep at this point. Some women are able to sleep through their early contractions, to get some much-needed rest to prepare for the birth, but I was wide awake. I sat on my favourite seat next to the kitchen window which overlooked Byres Road. I reminisced about all the conversations, parties and fun I'd had in the flat in years gone by. This was also where Gary and I had our first kiss. I realised that so much had changed in my life since those early days at college when I used to live there. And things were about to change for me again in a matter of hours when Gary and I would both become parents.

It was now 11.30pm. The pain was definitely intensifying now, enough to bring a few tears to my eyes in between contractions. I woke Gary who was fast asleep in the bedroom, grabbed my dressing gown and said, "If it's not time now, I don't think I'll survive this."

We drove the short journey back to the hospital. I was astonished to find out that I still wasn't fully dilated, but by this point my tears were enough to convince them to allow me up to the maternity floor. Gary and I clasped hands and walked through the long dark corridors of the hospital; it felt like we were caught in-between dreams. We passed a few delivery rooms on the way and could hear some grunts and noises from women in the throes of labour, followed by some softly spoken words of encouragement from their spouses. I was introduced to my midwife who would be with me until 6am the following morning, at which point she would hand me over to someone else if the baby hadn't arrived. I remember thinking that if the baby hadn't arrived by then I would gladly perform my own caesarean section! I checked myself out in the mirror and I thought I looked passably hot. I even felt for a second that I might miss my bump a little. I had a love–hate relationship with it. I didn't enjoy it accompanying me to parties or social events but it had become a great table for snacks and had got me to the front of many queues in recent months.

"Right, dear, here's what we're going to do. In this section here your baby will be born. Here is your birthing ball and some beanbags for your comfort. Move around as much as you like, it's good to keep active. This is your gas and air, which you can start now. Breathe in when you have a contraction. Try it."

I sucked on the pipe, but I didn't feel much effect straight away. I was a bit disappointed to say the least, so I asked the midwife if there was anything else I could try. She encouraged me to give it another go and after a few more tries I began to feel the effects. The gas part of the gas and air is nitrous oxide, otherwise known as laughing gas. As I started to giggle and feel slightly light-headed (perhaps a feeling I remember from my party nights), Gary thought it would be funny for him to have a go. Let's face it, he hadn't really been partying for nine months either. I took some big deep breaths of the gas and could feel that it was helping me calm down. Although it didn't take it away completely, it took the edge off the pain a little.

Gary took another couple of shots of the gas and air when the staff weren't looking and within minutes he was in stitches and decided to put a bed pan on his head to make me laugh. He was really getting into the whole experience, telling me that this was going to be a breeze. I hadn't seen him looking this uninhibited for around nine months. He was really cracking me up which also helped calm my nerves.

"I think my waters have broken," I yelped as I got up from bouncing on my ball.

It was game over. It looked like I hadn't had a pee in a year and it had just flowed out uncontrollably all over the floor. My sexy knee-high socks were ruined. Gary tried to pretend like he wasn't taken aback by what he was seeing but he wasn't doing a very good job, as his chin literally hit the floor. *Thank God he's high on gas and air,* I kept thinking.

"Run me a bath," I shouted, expecting a negative response. But by 7am I was relaxing in a warm bath, completely out of my mind on gas and air, pretending to be the fish out of *Finding Nemo*. Splashing around, pretending my arms were fins. What a sexy sight for Gary, I thought.

I was in unbearable pain as I tried to lift my legs over the bath to get transferred back through to my bed. I met my new midwife on the way in and realised I was now forty-plus hours into labour. I hadn't slept a wink and I was feeling exhausted now. How much longer would it take for my baby to come? The midwife had a good look at me and told me that a baby was in fact coming. It wasn't going to be long now. How could she see a baby up there? What was happening? Was I going to poop myself now? Would he leave me? I wanted a puppy; can somebody please just bring me a puppy?

I continued to practise my breathing techniques. The contractions were now at an unbearable level of intensity.

Gary's carefully chosen words of support and encouragement had really helped me stay positive throughout my labour experience, but the gas and air was the only thing helping to distract me from the pain and it somehow *ran out*. The midwives ran around looking for new canisters, shouting: "This has never happened before, this is unbelievable!" I turned around and witnessed a guilty look from Gary as he held my hand. He'd obviously taken a little bit too much of the gas and air.

As the staff set up another canister, the baby was well and truly making its way into the world. My God it hurt. I pushed, I screamed, I wanted to kill everyone in the room and most of all I just wanted a fucking puppy! But it was a baby I received.

A beautiful baby *boy*.

A tiny, wrinkly baby boy was held up in front of me as my Gary bravely cut the umbilical cord.

I just lay there astonished as I looked at my baby. I could hear the faint sounds of his innocent cries as the midwife placed my little boy upon my bare chest for skin-to-skin contact. The exhausting forty-six hour marathon of labour was now over and like some kind of miracle, I was holding a new life that Gary and I had created. As I held my newborn, I had an overwhelming sense of love that I believe you can only experience in this moment. All of my fears about how I was going to hold it together as a mother sort of evaporated. I knew in that perfect moment that I was going to fight like a mother lion to give my child everything I could give him. A light came on: it was not about me any more, it was all about him.

"You did it, you're amazing. Look at him, he is perfect," Gary said.

"Have you got a name for him?" the midwife who delivered my baby asked.

"Yes, we're calling him Oscar," I replied.

"Lovely name, my cat is called Oscar!" Good start, I thought. It was such a perfect coincidence.

Our little boy was now in the arms of his dad. I had just made my boyfriend a father. It was so beautiful. I was seeing him in a different light. I fell head over heels in love again, a much deeper love, a maternal love. The love of my life had exceeded all my expectations as my birthing partner. I knew as he held his son in his arms that this was the happiest moment of his life. It was written all over his face and I got to witness every moment. True love.

After a thorough examination from the midwife, as if giving birth isn't traumatising enough, I was then given an injection in my leg to *deliver my placenta* (yes, you need to push that out too – not at all sore though), and then I was invited to take a warm bath. I got the wrong end of the stick when I thought this was my opportunity to have a relaxing nap in the bath. I was awakened by a loud knock on the door after five minutes and I was told to get out to tend to my baby.

It had started.

Carrying my little bundle in my arms, I was taken in a wheelchair down to the ward. I was helped on to my bed and felt a sense of pride along with a slight feeling of insecurity as I looked around the room to realise that I most definitely was the youngest in that ward, by seven years at least. The midwives began to make their way around the ward, introducing themselves as they demonstrated how to change nappies and breastfeed. I was exhausted but fought against it in order to watch the demonstration and gave the midwife my full attention as she taught me how to feed Oscar. After around ten minutes, he was placed back in the basket beside me. I just stared. This seven-pound baby lay there so angelically. I wept for many hours, silently proud, silently scared but truly in love. He was just lying there helplessly, needing someone to love him, look after him, protect him. I had never felt this deep-rooted love before. I knew I could be a mother now. I knew that I would do anything for this small being with his long eyelashes, rosy cheeks and brown hair.

As the evening drew to a close, Gary left the ward and headed home. I reached into my bag for the free airliner sleeping mask that I had picked up and I slipped it over my eyes and looked forward to my night's sleep.

"Goodness, my dear, you can't use a sleeping mask now – you need to watch your baby," I heard a midwife gasp, as she rushed over to me.

In sheer panic I pulled back my mask, staring around the room and then relaxed to see that Oscar was still firmly wrapped up in his cot. All the other mothers were balancing their babies on their breasts in such a relaxed fashion that you would almost think they had given birth on a daily basis. A bout of deep shame overcame me. I'd only had my baby for a few hours and already I'd messed up. I drew the curtains around us both and looked at my phone to distract me. I opened it to a text message from my father that read: *Congratulations on your first OSCAR*.

I woke up the next morning in a panic. I heard trolleys, babies crying around me, doors opening and closing. I gazed at the clock on the wall. It was 6am and I had fallen asleep at 11pm after Oscar's feed. *Is he OK? Is he still alive?* And there he was, lying, wrapped so tightly in his blanket, sleeping peacefully. I wondered, *How, why? Have I slept through a full day?* The midwife on duty arrived at the side of my bed.

"How are you feeling?" she asked me, looking at me with her kind eyes.

"Really good, I can't believe I just slept right through, is he OK?"

"Yes dear, everything is fine; he is just tired too. He is beautiful."

"Thank you so much," I replied, trying not to cry.

"How big was he? You are so small," she asked.

"He was seven pounds two ounces."

"Good for you girl, how many stitches did you need?"

"None," I replied, and she gave a girl power high five. I obviously was really good at the pelvic floor exercises after all.

I felt slightly refreshed after six hours of uninterrupted bliss, though I was so swollen and sore as I sat up in bed and admired all the women in the room. All of us had different birth stories, and we each realised how lucky we were to have healthy babies. Although we were all at different stages in our lives, we were all going to be going through the exact same transition into motherhood.

I waited for the moment our families arrived to catch a glimpse of the Oscar we had created. I could hear them before I could see them. His new grandparents, aunties, uncles, cousins. They were all truly happy. We remained in hospital for two nights which gave me some more insight into how to change nappies, help my baby latch onto my breasts and how to keep him clean and healthy. I just couldn't wait to get him home.

The Third Trimester:

A summary of what's happening to you and your baby & the things I wish I had known

Congratulations! You've made it! You are now in the home stretch of your pregnancy – I told you it came in fast. Although the end is in sight, the third trimester is going to be the most uncomfortable of them all. The third trimester begins at week twenty-six until you give birth. Although you will have your due date, take this as an estimation, as your baby could come earlier or later! If you pass week forty of your pregnancy, you will be advised by your doctors of a date by which you will need to be induced into labour, usually around week forty-two.

Cool Things Happening This Month
- You'll begin your antenatal classes.
- You'll be finishing up in work.
- Most airlines won't let you fly past week thirty-five, so make sure any planned travel arrangements are discussed with your doctor.
- All your hard planning in the second trimester will be beginning to fall into place.
- As your baby continues to get bigger and stronger, you are bound to get kicked!
- Talk to your baby – he or she can hear you!
- You're actually going to give birth and meet your baby!

Antenatal Classes

Antenatal classes are a real blessing. Please go to them, as you will learn a lot! Classes typically take place during the third trimester, to teach you and your partner how best to prepare for labour, birth and early parenthood. It's a good idea if you can get your birthing partner (whether that's your partner, a friend, a parent) to attend these classes with you, to give you both confidence in what lies ahead. You will cover different areas, including pain relief, positions to assist in labour, breathing techniques, breastfeeding and how best to care for your baby once they come along. It's also the perfect time to ask lots of questions and speak to all the other mothers in the room. Sometimes people make life-long friends in these classes.

Your Body

- Belly button – Even if you have an 'innie', you are likely to develop an 'outie' as your baby grows. It does make some outfits look strange!
- Nipples – Your nipples may begin to change in size and shape, more so towards the end of your pregnancy. Lumpy, darker, bigger nipples are all normal. Nipples change for the reason that it makes it easier for your baby to latch on. Don't be concerned at the changes; they are just doing their job!
- Hunger games – As your pregnancy progresses you may feel like you can't eat the full birthday cake you did at week twelve. This is due to the baby taking up most of the room in there, so be sure to eat smaller, easier meals. However, during the third trimester it is recommend, to eat only an extra 200 calories a day (of the good stuff!).
- Breathing – It's not uncommon to have a shortness of

breath at this point in pregnancy, again thanks to all the extra pressure of a growing baby. It might be at times hard to catch your breath; however, this should only be with exertion – any unusual shortness of breath must be checked out, especially if unprovoked by physical activity.

Breasts getting ready for feeding

Along with your bump, your breasts will be growing larger by the week preparing to produce milk for when the baby comes. During this trimester, you may experience some leaking yellow custardy fluid from your nipples. This is called colostrum, the precursor to your breastmilk that contains more protein and less sugar and fat, making it easier for your baby to digest. This is what baby will feed on until your breastmilk comes in. Colostrum is also full of antibodies, which can help your baby fight infection.

- If you have not experienced any leaking – yet are curious – try squeezing your areola to see it; however, not everyone can see this!
- Everyone's colostrum comes at different times, so don't worry if you don't experience it.
- If you are experiencing leaks, now is the time to begin your journey with breast pads (more about these later!).

Braxton Hicks

Braxton Hicks contractions are something to be aware of, and can sometimes come on in the second trimester. They were something I always looked out for, but they never happened to me personally. They feel like contractions, and they should happen infrequently and they should be painless. They are warm-up contractions preparing your uterus for the labour that lies ahead.

Signs to call your doctor:

- The contractions are getting closer together.
- They are happening on a regular basis.
- You are out of breath at the end of the contractions.

Baby Brain

I really hope you have a sense of humour, because you are really going to need it at some points during this trimester! If you have ever heard of people feeling like they have 'brain fog', well, you might be in line to experience this soon. As much as our pregnancy hormones like to give us various problems, they too like to have a bit of fun so get ready to become a bit more forgetful! That is why it's good to have a diary, or set reminders on your phone with all your upcoming appointments you don't want to miss. Don't worry, your brain will bounce back soon!

Other People's Opinions

In the third trimester as you begin to stand out from the crowd, you may now elicit a few concerned looks from various members of your community. It's likely also that people will begin to touch your growing baby (whether you like it or not!) and comment things like: "Aww, you have a massive bump, do you think it will be around ten pounds?" or "Are you really eight months pregnant? Your bump is so small." – any opportunity to add to the anxiety.

- Let them stare, just smile back, confuse them all!
- Be polite – because they are all just trying to be nice in the end and congratulate you.
- Everyone will have a story to tell you about their own

pregnancy, how sore labour is, how their child didn't sleep for two years, how awful their stretch marks are now – you can't filter conversations, but you can choose what you let in.

Planning Ahead

Now is the time to start thinking about tying up all the loose ends you didn't manage to in the second trimester. Organise a food shop for before the baby comes and get your freezer stocked up with some food and welcome some home-cooking from parents to pop in there too! Make sure that you have a car seat fitted safely – this is so important for your journey home from the hospital.

Birthing Plan

Yes, darling, that baby is coming out of you. Having a birth plan is something that will be covered in your antenatal classes, and unlike me, it may be something you would like to give a bit of thought to. To my knowledge, not many mothers successfully accomplish all their goals on their birthing plans, but if anything it should help you and your midwife to understand your expectations, give you a chance to explore options and give you and idea of what you are in for! A birthing plan is a way for you to communicate to your midwife and medical team on the day how you would like to deliver and how you want to manage pain relief. Remember, midwives don't work twenty-four hours, so even though you may have become attached to the nice lady that runs the antenatal class, it doesn't mean she will be there to deliver your baby. So providing a document, which you may receive from an antenatal class, to the midwife looking after you is a step in the right direction. Make sure you ask and understand what pain relief might be open to you if you decide to give birth in hospital or in the comfort of your own home. Know that there are options open to you, so again this is just another decision you will need to make. Many hospitals and clinics will have tailored birthing plan spreadsheets available for you to take home, discuss with your partner and bring with you to labour.

Include in Your Hospital Bag

You will not know how long you are going to be in hospital for once baby comes along so it's best to stock up on the following items to see you through a minimum of two nights. Your family can always bring you extras if you need.

For you

- Dressing gown
- Two pairs of cotton pyjamas
- Slippers
- Changes of underwear
- Nursing bra
- Breasts pads (at least two packs)
- Sanitary towels
- Face wipes
- Make-up
- Comfortable day clothes
- Snacks – something tasty!
- Bottles of water
- Mobile phone charger
- Camera
- TENS machine (can assist with pain during labour)
- Going-home outfit
- A favourite lotion or something that will soothe you
- Your birthing plan
- Loose change in case there's a decent vending machine

For your baby

- Sleeping suits
- An outfit for going home (weather appropriate)
- Nappies
- Wipes
- Blankets
- A new car seat to take your baby home in – make sure it is fitted correctly
- If you are not choosing to breastfeed, remember bottles

Labour

Did you just skip the book and come straight to this section? I don't blame you. Pregnancy is a daunting process which leads up to the inevitable final push. I have not spoken to two mums who tell me a similar labour story, everyone's is unique, but I hope for you, that it is blissfully easy. If your labour comes on naturally, there are three common signs to look out for.

- Lower back or abdominal pain that won't go away, like menstrual feelings and cramps.
- Painful contractions or feelings of tightening that may be irregular in strength and frequency and may stop and start.
- Your waters break (this can feel different for everyone – but you will know).
- Legs might begin to cramp up.
- You may feel very sick with all the sensations as your body prepares to deliver your baby.

First-time mums can be in early labour for many hours, sometimes going into days. You may begin by feeling shorter and infrequent cramps, which is just your body getting prepared. If you find yourself in a long, early labour, like I did, here are some tips on things to do to pass the time:

- Go for a nice walk in the fresh air – not alone though!
- Listen to your favourite album.
- Get your final pamper package sorted.
- Start to do your relaxing breathing techniques that they taught you in class.

When you arrive at the hospital, a nurse or doctor will evaluate you to see how far on you are in labour. This is a good time to discuss your birthing plan, as you enter into the first phase of active labour. You will be settled in to your room and can begin your real labour journey by trying to get as comfortable as possible! The final stage of labour can take anywhere between a few minutes and an hour, once you are dilated enough and have the urge to push your baby out. Once its head is out, its body will follow and you will begin to feel a great sense of relief.

During the third stage of labour you will deliver the placenta. This will be a lot less painful and can take up to thirty minutes to do. You will feel less painful contractions and be asked to push it out at the right time. There will then be an inspection to see if you need any stitches; if so, this will be done there and then and you can move on from it all very quickly and start getting to know your baby.

It's all worth it. Promise!

Back to You

As you come closer to the end of your pregnancy, you might begin to feel overwhelmed with worry that you won't be up to the role of mother, that you're still not ready. Trust me, you are. Life will be consumed with looking after your new baby, so now is the time to reflect, spend some time doing the things you enjoy and start writing down a list of things that you want to achieve once baby is here. It can be as simple as 'I want to fit back into my jeans' or it could be 'I want to be a successful actress' – give yourself some goals and write them down. Time moves quickly, and you need to stay focused on you. My mother told me to spend my final few days as a free young mum-to-be doing things I loved. Visiting art galleries, stuffing myself with popcorn in the movies, going to watch a play. It was one of the best bits of advice I got at this stage of pregnancy, so take it!

Your Baby's Growth in the Third Trimester

Your baby will be gaining weight rapidly over this time, moving a lot more, while your body is making a lot of final touches to its development. By the end of the third trimester your baby will be ready to enter the world. It's worth remembering that your baby may come early or late. If your baby arrives prematurely, before the end of month seven, he or she will be taken to special care, but will likely be able to come home after a few weeks.

Weeks 25–28

Your baby is beginning to deposit fat. It is also around the size of a cauliflower head! Your baby can now fully hear everything and is moving into various positions. Your baby is now able to respond to light, pain and sound.

Weeks 29–32

Your baby is now around eight inches long and will weigh around five pounds. Your baby is continuing to develop fat reserves. The brain is developing rapidly during this month and you will definitely feel some more kicks and people will be able to feel them too! Although most of baby's internal systems are well developed, its lungs are still developing at this stage.

Weeks 33–40

Your baby is getting ready for its exit – and is continuing to grow by the day; it will be around the length of a stalk of rhubarb! His or her lungs will now be fully developed. If this is going to be your first baby it will hopefully be getting into position for labour and drop down to your pelvis usually with its head pointed down towards the birth canal.

Shopping List for YOU During the Third Trimester
- A support band for your growing bump
- Nursing bras and tops
- Breast pads to help your leaking breasts
- Extra-comfy clothing
- Trainers
- Pregnancy massage
- New bedding for yourself; you may begin to leak milk
- TENS machine

Shopping List for your BABY During the Third Trimester
- A car seat – this needs to be new and safe
- A stroller/pram
- A Moses basket for your baby to sleep in by your bed for the first few months
- Bedding for your baby's bed – and a few spares – you may need to change everyday
- If you are deciding to bottle feed, bottles and milk

PS

You are going to meet your baby soon! As you progress through this trimester, just know that no one finds it easy. If I can give you one bit of advice at this point, it's to have a sense of humour about it. Sometimes you just have to laugh. Take some time for you and don't leave everything until the last minute, because your baby really could come any time now!

Reflections

I'd never had to deal with a death like this before. I was having to allow myself to be vulnerable when I was trying my best to be strong for baby and everyone around me. It was really strange going through death and birth within such a short period of time.

I was thirteen when I found out my uncle was going to die. Old enough to know what it meant, but definitely not old enough to appreciate that life had a timeframe. Five years seemed like ages away; like, I'd just be leaving school, and what a drag that thought was. I was on automatic at thirteen: eyeliner, crop tops, hair styles, flared trousers and high boots were the most important factor in my life. I thought I had my whole life ahead of me. But how could life just be cut short like that? I thought, *How is that fair?* I think by the time our pregnancy came along, I knew this all too well. I knew I might not have another chance. I'd found out the hard way how fragile life was.

As Ernest Hemingway put it: "Every man's life ends the same way. It is only the details of how he lived and how he dies that distinguish one man from another."

He'd set an example to me. He had also taught me that if I couldn't be strong in life, well, I best be brave. He wanted to be on this planet for every last second he could be, which taught me how precious life was. He was a man in his early fifties who wished he could have had even five minutes longer with us, when he should have really had another forty years at least. There was so much to look forward to in life, and we needn't waste it on over worrying, analysing or doubting ourselves, we should just be out there living it.

Perhaps this was one of the reasons why I just went for my driver's licence. It maybe should have been way down in my priority lists at that point, but having a licence seemed to be confirmation to me that I could mother (we all have our own reasons why we do things). It did prove to me yet again that once you put your mind to something, once you put your wishes out there, sometimes the universe will listen. Don't get me wrong, I've asked the universe for lots of things, including an extra two inches of height and an extra box of spicy Peperamis, and nothing appeared. But I'd planned for that test, and I decided to be brave. It worked out for me.

Labour in the end was one of the most magical experiences I will ever have. It was utterly breathtaking. I will never forget it, for none of the sore parts. Why should something so beautiful not be worth a bit of pain? Don't we all go through a bit of pain to get something that we really want or love? Even in our working lives, in managing our relationships, even in the things we want to be good at. I could have laid on that bed for hours weeping tears of sheer joy and amazement once Oscar was delivered. Nothing prepared me for the feelings I was experiencing, or how the thoughts in my head changed from *How am I going to survive this* to *I am one of the lucky ones who get to experience this*.

Labour changed my mindset on my body. I'd spent months trying to learn how to look after it as it grew, but I never for a second appreciated it like I did in those moments. I couldn't quite understand how all of this growth and development happened inside me and how our bodies just know what to do to bring our babies out. I still don't know if I can sum it up. It was by far one of the greatest experiences of my life.

I was lucky to experience something like this early on in life, because in turn, it made me appreciate my body more and it taught me to see through all the changes that happened to me throughout pregnancy and be grateful for it for giving me a healthy baby. How could I be so hard on myself when I just managed to do all of this? This experience gave me more belief in myself than I ever had before. I couldn't quite get how I'd managed to go through all of that. But you just do. It's like second nature.

And as I held my baby in my arms, I knew that it wasn't just the beginning for him, but the beginning for me. I'd now accepted who I was, for what I was, and all I wanted to be, was his mother.

PART 4

Nappy Time into Early Motherhood

Welcome Home, Baby

It'll be the first night that we had spent in the new home that we had been preparing for months. There was a sense of peace in the air. Our new home still smelled of freshly laid carpets, fresh paint and with a distinct aroma of all the fresh flowers that had been delivered. We walked into our home, carrying the baby in his car seat as though we held the crown jewels. We placed him down on the sitting room floor and just stared. He was so much smaller than we had been expecting, so fragile. I wondered about how it must have felt for him being out in the world, with all the new smells, sounds and sensations. I guess I was going to experience all that too.

My maternal instincts had kicked in and I was going to protect this little baby, my baby, for ever. I had a new love in my life. There was an unfamiliar sense of calmness within me that I had never felt before. The role I was taking on, which before had seemed so alien, was now a centre of stillness where everything fell into place. I found myself to be completely in tune with motherhood.

We had spent weeks preparing the most beautiful crib by the bed, looking forward to the day we would have a baby lying in there. You could prepare your home with lots of wonderful new expensive gadgets and furniture, but believe me: they are not appreciated by your baby. Oscar spent his first few nights in his pram getting wheeled around in the darkened sitting room until he finally settled. It wasn't until night three that we managed to get him to settle in the crib by the bed, and it wasn't the crying that was keeping me up, it was the most peculiar animal sounds that were coming out of him! It was a cacophony of sounds and it made us both laugh, a lot. There was something very special about the fact that I could just pick him up and he could feed while I was lying in my cosy bed. I just wanted to nurture him, to make him feel safe and loved.

Nothing prepared me for the intensity of the first few weeks as I was getting to know him. It was more than a full-time job – it was my entire life. The early days were like waking up in the middle of a dream, confused as to where I was and they were also relentlessly busy with breastfeeding, nappy changing, bathing, winding, sleeping and also visits from family, neighbours and friends. Healthcare visits from our local midwife were so essential. I looked forward to her knocking on the door so that I could have a good old moan about how sore my boobs were, how tired I was, how the baby would not settle, how my house was never going to be clean again, how Gary needed to go back to work tomorrow and it would just be baby and me all day long.

Days turned into nights, each day bringing a new sound, a new movement, a smile. I was falling so in love with moments. Moments of seeing Gary lie next to him, so at peace, adapting to his new role as father. I was beginning to take a step back and look at the miracle of life from afar, from a perspective I'd never had before. A deeper love and connection was formed with the guy I had fallen so madly in love with only a year before. Our love really had gone the distance here and I was lucky to feel so secure and loved as we both morphed into this new chapter of being parents.

A new-found appreciation for my mother, for all mothers out there continued to develop within me, mothers whose lives are turned upside down yet they stay committed to giving their children everything. I was so, so grateful for *Mad Men* and box sets. The outside world seemed too fast to keep up with now.

As we continued to make finishing touches to our home, I took time out to go in search for a TV. I realised quickly that I would be spending a lot more time indoors, getting to know my baby, so some extra entertainment was very much appreciated. As I walked alone around the electrical shop a gentleman who worked there came up to me.

"Can I help you with anything?" he asked.

"Yes, I'm looking for a TV for my house," I replied.

His eyes were now stationed on my breasts, which made me feel rather awkward. I knew they were impressive, but his eyes kept opening wider and wider until his jaw almost hit the floor.

"Are you OK?" he asked, casually pointing to my breasts.

I looked down at my white top and realised I had had a major leak. Both nipple areas were soaked through and had produced two wide, wet, drooping circles. It was horrific. I hurriedly left the shop and scrambled through the changing bag for something to cover myself with, and something to help with the stench roaring from my top. Milk had leaked through a set of breast pads confirming to me that I would need to double them up from this point on. I think I must have put the poor retail assistant off boobs for life, the poor guy.

As Gary was now to return to work I began to wonder if it was time to draw up some courage and make my way to the local mums' coffee morning in the village. After weeks of battling with myself and wishing that Oscar would have more babies to interact with I eventually got myself together and made my way around. I hadn't felt nerves like this since before going on stage. I was going to have to become the character of a mumsy mum in order to be accepted into the group. But

I was eager to make friends in this new town where we based ourselves, friends that I would have something in common with. As I pulled into the car park, the coffee shop window was all steamed up. I could see a few heads moving. It looked busy. As I pulled the door back to enter, awkwardly carrying my ten-week-old baby in his car seat, I scanned the room and caught sight of what I dreaded most: women in their thirties, exposed breasts, feeding their children proudly and gasping about how well they had slept last night, how well their babies were latching on, and how the midwife was so delighted with their progress. I walked straight to the counter.

"Can I have a coffee to go, please? I need to get to an appointment," I said nervously.

Needless to say no one looked in my direction. I thought they must have been hoping that I wouldn't sit down and say hello, as if they would be the mortified ones. I could tell within five seconds that this local group would only fill me with more anxiety over the job I was still unsure of, and decided that groups like this weren't really going to help me after all. I was closing that door.

It was always me and my baby. Whether he was sleeping in his Moses basket while I bathed, attached to my chest with a sling while I cleaned the house, while I went to the toilet, while I fed him. There was no break, no time to think about what I wanted or enjoyed, or who I was. I was slowly, but surely, losing my old self, I was just a mum now.

We realised quickly that if we wanted to make time for each other as a couple, it was going to take a lot of careful planning and execution, but we kept to our promise to continue our Friday night movie date. However, from now on it took place from the comfort of our own home.

"Let's pour some wine, stick on some music and get ready

to head out on the town. Let's go to that movie that's just come out and then afterwards go to our favourite club that plays really good rock 'n' roll, and dance until the club closes and just follow the crowd to whatever party we end up at. Tomorrow we can wake up, throw some clothes on and wander into town, browse the shops and have a nice lunch somewhere. Then, let's come home, go for a nap, watch Netflix and open up that expensive bottle of wine that I got for my birthday," said no parents in the first few months of parenthood. Ever.

As the weeks went by and we got Oscar into a routine, we allowed the grandparents to babysit for the night. They took Oscar out which meant Gary and I had the place all to ourselves. We should have probably thought about christening all the rooms in our new house now that we were both alone. I nipped upstairs and made myself more presentable, you know, took my hair tie out and wriggled my hair a little. I then took my slippers off so my unpainted toes were on show. I spent a few minutes considering whether or not to put on a dress before realising I hadn't shaved my legs for two months. I decided to keep my leggings on. I considered putting on some make-up until I decided that that would take too long and a little bit of lip gloss would do. All I really wanted to be doing was enjoying our date night.

I went downstairs to be greeted by the man of my dreams, in his work clothes, fast asleep on the couch, remote control in hand. Heaven.

I let him sleep and went through to fill the dishwasher. I then began to sterilise some bottles and play some nursery music in the background, to set the scene. Once the kitchen was clean, I moved on to the living room and tidied up for the fifth time that day, but not before checking in with the grandparents to make sure Oscar was OK. I then emptied the nappy bin just to add to the charm of the romantic night that lay ahead. The scene was set.

Once the house was ready I whispered in my lover's ear, "Let's go to the bedroom," and he just lay there, completely unresponsive. I turned down the lights and made my way upstairs alone. I decided to slip into something sexy, like a pair of boxers, and rummaged for the only T-shirt that wasn't covered in baby milk and shit. I then climbed into bed and breathed a sigh of relief, before turning off the lights after three whole minutes of considering whether or not to read or watch trash TV. I began to drift off and spent that night waking up every three hours wondering how Oscar was. Gary made his way up to the bedroom in the middle of the night and lay down next to me whispering something sexy in my ear like, "Night night." We drifted back to sleep, and rose after a 'long lie-in' until 6am surrounded by a damp patch on the bed from my leaking breasts, and the scent of soured milk lingering in the air. I took off my T-shirt and sat on the edge of the bed expressing milk out of my swollen breasts. He started to rub my back, and said something beautiful like, "Oh, they look really sore."

Early months of motherhood were a whirlwind.

Nappy Time:

A summary of what's happening to you and your baby & the things I wish I had known

Motherhood comes with its own set of teething problems, including those that need Bonjela, Sophie the Giraffe and hundreds and thousands of warm cuddles. This was no Tamagotchi or fake doll that you take home from school to see if you can cope with a small baby. It's a twenty-four-hour job, and it's all down to you. You have now become a slave to the baby and it becomes the centre of your universe. There is nothing harder or nothing sweeter. Slowly but surely you get to know each other and life settles into a routine that will help to restore some time back to you for tasks needing done, or a well earned rest. All the hard work is paying off.

You will be having health visits in the comfort of your home. This is the chance to ask lots of questions, seek help and soak up all the advice you are given for your growing baby.

Body Changes

Belly

After birth you may continue to look pregnant for up to seven weeks or longer. Although your uterus shrinks back into your pelvis, your abdominal muscles get stretched out during pregnancy and it will take time, eating correctly and exercise to get your belly back in shape. Your brown line will disappear, but your stretch marks may stick around – even celebrities have them, but they also have access to great Photoshop, so don't compare yourself. OK? Good! You might need to work a bit harder to get rid of the bulge, but only you can make it happen, so get crunching.

Cinderella moment

Yes, if you have suffered from any swelling during pregnancy this should be on its way out and you'll be able to fit nicely into all your old shoes in no time (shame it's not this easy with your favourite jeans).

Hair

You may notice that your hair will begin to fall out. During pregnancy, as you know, your hair grows at a faster pace and doesn't fall out. But once your baby is out, expect this to fall out too. Don't worry though, soon your hair will return to its normal cycle growth.

Skin

If you suffered from acne or dry skin during pregnancy, expect this to begin to disappear over the early weeks of motherhood. Take good care of your skin though as it begins to bounce back.

Breast changes

Now that your baby is out and you may be preparing for breastfeeding, your breasts will become more swollen and sore, and may start leaking milk in the first few days. The swelling will come down in the coming days as you start breastfeeding. If you are not intending to breastfeed you may still leak milk for up to seven weeks, so always wear breast pads.

Sweating

Although you can experience a lot of sweating throughout your pregnancy, it might feel more like a problem after giving birth. This primarily happens at night-time and is caused by your body trying to rid itself of all the extra fluids it accumulated during the pregnancy.

Constipation

If you haven't experienced constipation yet, you may as you enter into the first weeks of motherhood. For me, I was so scared of going to the toilet anyway that it just didn't happen. I'm also not sure if I ate much in the first few weeks, it was all a bit hazy.

Will my vagina ever be the same again?

No one warns you about the aftermath of having a baby, or how sore you are down below. Perhaps people are too embarrassed to speak out about it, but I did tell you this book was honest, so why stop now? If you have a natural vaginal birth expect to sting, shout, laugh and cry when you take a pee for two weeks afterwards. My first pee after giving birth can only be described as someone placing boiling hot, prickly coal on my flower. I leaned over the sink trying not to be sick after my first attempt. *Ouchy!* I told you motherhood's a bitch, right?

I resorted to various tactics to lessen the torture:

- Spray cold water on that area using a shower head.
- Stock up on frozen peas and ice cubes.
- Drink only water.
- Keep doing your pelvic floor exercises and regain your former tone!

The pain will begin to subside over the coming weeks. I promise. The periods you haven't had for the past nine months may also be something to get used to again, as you will notice blood and what is left of your uterine lining (lochia) of your pregnancy show up in place of the discharge you have been experiencing. Vaginal bleeding after birth can last up to six weeks and can vary in colour throughout that time. Following on from this your periods may become irregular as your body gets used to not having a baby in it to develop, so be patient with yourself and your body.

Let's Talk About SEX Again

After getting over my first few weeks of being unable to urinate without screaming, I was moving towards the day this was going to happen with great caution. I was worried I may never want to again, that I would always be too tired, too lazy to involve in any extra-curricular activity. We had not long passed our one-year anniversary together, so we were still in the honeymoon of our relationship, so sex was certainly at the forefront of my mind a lot, but would he want to have sex with me and my new body? *Yes*. As you quickly adapt to your role as a mother, your partner might find it quite sexy. Most likely *not* always your appearance (I've never seen a Kim Kardashian playing her motherhood role go viral), but the way you are with your child, what you can tolerate, the person you have become, they are seeing you in a completely new light and this may be pretty hot!

As the day approaches, what might help?

- A glass of Prosecco to ease the fears.
- Leave it six weeks until everything is working again (if you can – if you want to go for it earlier, check with your doctor – not Google).

- Make sure you are using contraception – unless you want to go through all this again.
- Keep your bra on with some breast pads in – leaking over him might not be sexy.
- Don't worry about your body if it's not back to the way you want it. You've just carried a child around in there for nine months and delivered it – how HOT is that?

Breastfeeding

Everyone will have their own unique experience of breastfeeding.

I wanted to be that confident mother in Starbucks, balancing a feeding baby on one arm while reading a book on how to be the best mother on the other. The mother who is drinking green tea, accepting compliments from the passers-by and just sitting there, proud and strong in her new-found role. I wanted to feel proud of my body. I wanted to ooze with confidence and milk. I wanted to feel less embarrassed about all the change that had happened. "Breast is best, breast is best" were words that kept going around in my fragile head space. I think the word 'breastfeeding' was uddered – I mean, *uttered* – to me before anybody asked when the baby was due. I got to grips with the fact that it was an essential part of caring for the baby as best I possibly could. My breasts had surprised me. My flat chest had blossomed into two perfectly rounded camel humps and I was hopeful that they would stick around (as was my boyfriend.) I felt too insecure to just whip them out in public though, so breastfeeding for me was filled with a few anxieties. But just like all mothers, you become second priority and baby is first, so I knew I was going to give it my best shot. A few reasons why breastfeeding is a good idea:

- Breastmilk contains antibodies which help newborns fight infection and decreases the chance of allergies.
- Breastfeeding is known to help decrease your chances of developing breast or ovarian cancer.
- Physical contact will help you bond with baby.
- Breastfeeding burns a lot of calories.
- It will save you money.

To get off to the best start with breastfeeding:
- Keep your baby skin-to-skin as much as possible after birth.
- Remember that your baby knows how to latch on – their face needs to be in contact with the breast so that they can figure out where to latch on.
- Get help sooner rather than later – midwives and local support groups will help you as much as you need with beginning your breastfeeding journey.

Don't get me wrong – it's not always easy. The early days when you are exhausted and you are trying to get baby to latch on your sore nipples can make you feel like giving up real quick. I thought pushing him out was bad enough but fuck me, this took the biscuit. That said, feeding Oscar was one of the most beautiful experiences about the early days, as it gave me the chance to connect with him and comfort him. On reflection, I should have asked for more help, asked the midwife to come back to my hospital bed and spend more time with me until I felt confident in what I was doing. I also should have been that confident mother in Starbucks, because there was nothing for me to be embarrassed about. Breastfeeding is wonderful.

Maintaining Relationships

If you can bring a child into the world with the support of grandparents, you are lucky. For all the difference of opinions, for all the unannounced visits, for all the crushing love they bring, they will be your greatest support network and you will need them as much as the baby needs you. But remember, they had children too – you're one of them! So with the support also comes the lectures about the *'right way'* and *'this is what I did and my children turned out fine'*, which may influence how you bring up your own. We all have different opinions on the right way to bring up a child, but it's worth remembering that there is quite simply no manual; there is no right or wrong way. We cannot perfect parenthood. Just as you think you are perfecting one part of motherhood, your child changes. You are constantly adapting to your daily-changing child who is growing alongside their needs, so don't worry if your way is perceived as different; you will know what's best for your child.

Teamwork

You may find yourself wanting to take 100 per cent responsibility for absolutely everything your baby needs. Your motherly instincts will have kicked in and the thought of someone else changing his nappy or cradling him to sleep doesn't cross your mind, because you want to do everything for your child. Of course this is natural, but you will become exhausted over time. Ask your partner to take over for a while and rest up. Sleep while the baby sleeps during the day. Don't worry about whether or not the dinner is made or the washing machine is on.

Together alone

I would be lying if I told you I didn't want to be at the pool parties with my sister in Vancouver, or down in London doing a film course with Sadie, or drinking beer with my brother in Thailand, or starting university with my sister in Glasgow, or leaving school with options like my youngest sister. At times, I would have done anything to swap, even for a day, for one hour, to feel that sense of freedom, the sense of me, to breathe, to know again what it feels like to have the world at your feet. To know how it sounds to listen to a song without it being interrupted with tears, to read a book without having to change a nappy a few chapters in, to have friends all around me again on that dance floor. Anything rather than being in that house, just the two of us, all day long. There were times when I felt like a prisoner in my home, knowing all the while that outside the world kept revolving. Everyone warned me of how tiring motherhood could be, but no one mentioned the word lonely once. Motherhood can be a lonely game at times.

- You might feel like you don't fit into a certain group, or baby club, but everyone has gone through their own pregnancy, everyone will be getting used to their new life. Take comfort in the fact that however old or insecure you are, we are all human and new mothers more than anyone know the importance of companionship.
- What do you enjoy? We can so easily forget what we used to be interested in but pick up your hobbies and get reacquainted with your interests. You are important too and it's key to make some time for yourself, even if it's just booking yourself a massage. It's the least you deserve!
- Stay positive – there is light at the end of the tunnel! Yes, I hear you say, "It's easy for you to say, you're writing a book – blah blah blah!" Even getting to the point where I could put this book together came with much

frustration, fear and disappointments. I wish I was more positive and believed in myself sooner, so please do, you will be wonderful at whatever you put your mind to outside your parenting duties.

Your Child's Development in the First Few Months

Although the days will go by so quickly as you settle down to your new life with your baby, your baby will be continuing to develop outside of the womb and will astonish you in the coming weeks. Your baby will most likely cry a lot in the early days as he or she learns to communicate with you and slowly you will get into a routine and settle into motherhood. Each child develops at their own pace, so be patient and raise any concerns you may have.

In the first few months your baby is still getting used to the outside world. They will be responding to your voice and their eyesight will become fully developed. Your baby will now begin giving you an array of facial expressions, including smiles. Your baby will be beginning to hold their own head up and using their hands a lot to hold and play and feel their surroundings. Their hand and eye coordination are developing and their eyes will be following you around the room to make sure you don't go too far away!

Your baby will become fully engaged from four months onwards as he or she begins to laugh and have attempts at conversations. Your baby may also try to communicate through their hands and facial expressions. Don't worry, you'll definitely know if something is upsetting them! Your baby will start trying to sit up by themselves and become more mobile as they begin to shuffle around, rolling back and fourth on their tummy. It's now time to instil a bit of discipline, as your not-so-little baby is beginning to adjust to what they can get away with. They can now sense the tone in your voice, so they begin to understand that when Mummy says, 'No,' she means *No!* Your baby will also start responding to their name now and you will continue, day by day, to fall more in love with moments.

PS

You made it! Thank you for coming along for the ride. Becoming a parent, at any age, opens up the opportunity to grow, so embrace it! I know, you can't even remember what life was like before you had a baby – did you really have all that free time? If you're like me, you're only realising now how much you wish you hadn't wasted it. No book can properly prepare you for motherhood, not even this one. (Do you like how I left this until the end?) You can read all the books about pregnancy and motherhood, but in the end everyone's journey is different and how we cope with our new lives varies, so never feel like you are the only mother in the world who makes mistakes. You are not alone.

Reflections

I realised that I was a bit of an introvert during pregnancy, which meant being in the house or walking outside just the two of us was good enough for me. I could live without the coffee mornings or the mother/baby yoga. I wasn't a bad mother because of it. Looking back, I think had I pushed myself even further out of my comfort zone, loneliness would not have played such a big part. Perhaps I should have tried harder to look for young mums I had something in common with, because there are so many out there. Or maybe I should have felt less different to the other mothers and sat down with them and put all my insecurities aside. Alas, I am human, but I know now how rewarding it can be to surround yourself with other mothers, so put yourself out there – only good can come of it.

I can't say that parenthood was harder than I was expecting, because when it's your child, it doesn't seem hard. Trust me, I never in my wildest dreams thought I would go 'awwww' when Oscar broke wind, or clean up poop without feeling sick, or happily stay up all night just to make sure he was safe. Everything just fell into place organically when he came along. It's a real pleasure to be his mother.

I spent a lot of time worrying throughout my pregnancy that I was never going to figure out what my life had in store for me. I became filled with anxiety that I would never find my 'purpose' in life, that all I was going to be was a mother. As if that wasn't good enough. But something changed within me when I gave birth and spent the first few months with Oscar. I began to feel that just being a mother was good enough.

Do you even remember me? The girl who couldn't make a bowl of soup? Who didn't have a job, a ring on my finger or a tidy house? Who wasn't sure if she was ready to be a mum? The girl who was so lost and anxious about what her life may turn out like, a girl overwhelmed?

Well, she grew up a little bit.

I obviously learned a lot from my young years pretending to be a hotel receptionist at the local hotel, because that's the first job I landed when I went back to work when Oscar was seven months old. It never crossed my mind that I would just be a receptionist again – I was meant to be a famous actress, remember! But I was so much more than a receptionist now, so much more than the long shift hours, so much more than the minimum wage. How many jobs wake you up smiling? How many jobs offer you rewards like witnessing your baby take its first steps, opening its mouth for its first taste of solids? How many jobs give you a sense of real deep purpose? How many jobs pay you in love not money? How many jobs challenge you to be a better human, to be kinder, smarter, to be the person that someone really admires?

I'd landed the dream job without even knowing it. I wasn't just a part-time receptionist. I was a mum. No other job in the world could ever fulfil me in the way that this little boy does. I was growing up alongside this little baby, challenging myself every day to be a better human, to take care of him the best I could and to strive daily to give him the best life. I wasn't going to get dismissed from this role no matter how many mistakes I made along the way.

As I got to grips with motherhood, I realised that it didn't matter one bit that I was 'only' nineteen. We all worry about our futures regardless of our status. We are all at the exact same stage when we become pregnant and then mothers. We all have to adapt and learn at the same time. This isn't a job you need a good CV for, Louboutins, a good car, a Silver Cross pram – bloody hell, you don't even need a partner! I've met so many amazing single mothers and fathers along my way in parenthood who complain even less than I do at times. Everyone is doing their best. Parenthood is exactly what you make of it.

Be the change you want to see in the world!

What better way to do that than through your own children? Raising them to be kinder and stronger, so that the world is filled with hope for the future. We can't always get it right. But as long as we try, we're further than we have ever been.

And as I settled into my transition into motherhood, witnessing every day the beauty of Oscar, my new life meant I would often think of the man who never once judged our position. A man who accepted me for exactly who I was. The first person to tell us that we were going to be great parents. My uncle. He just knew. The journey with him made me far stronger and empowered me to become the best mother that I could be and to appreciate, through challenging days, that I, we, are very lucky to be here.

And now? Well, I'm still a bit messy. I still like to dance on tables from time to time. I still have the desire to move to New York one day to finish my acting training. I still have a bit of a potty mouth when Oscar's not around. I still cook terrible meals at times. I'm still a bit of a dreamer. But that is who I am.

I will always be improving.

But if there is anything I am sure of, it's that I'm a really good mother. Just like you'll be. And by the way, being a mother is the best thing in the world. I would take nappy time over party time, every time.

Dear Reader,

My journey is not unique. It's real, it's honest and it's written for you. Life as a parent will never be the same for you. Life will only become better, fuller, richer and most definitely more rewarding. Young motherhood is an adventure that I never saw myself being on, but it has taken me on the greatest journey so far, and through all the highs, lows and insecurities that you might face in your pregnancy, and through all the early days of sheer exhaustion which follow when baby arrives. Life was slowly but surely replaced by one with more energy, more humour and definitely more joy.

Don't feel inadequate because you feel scared, or lonely, or beaten, or because you have to reach out for support. You are not alone. It's the struggle that makes it all worthwhile and although we are now wearing the cape of a super-hero mum, we are still human, with feelings, with ambition, with our own personal needs. Let the love carry you through – and that might just be the love between you and your child because someone wasn't up for the role of father, but that is okay too. Just keep looking forward. You'll be fine.

So log off the Internet, stop worrying about the other people, and start focusing on you. Spend more time outside, breathing in the fresh air, being present to the miracle that is life itself. Carry this book with you, and pass it on to one of the thousands of expectant mothers who might need this more than you, sitting alone in a coffee shop, wishing they were part of something. Find that thing that you want to be part of, something that makes you feel like you again, and don't give up until you've got you back.

I promise you this. You will go on to surprise yourself. You are more capable than anyone ever thought you were, more capable than even you knew you were. And you are now the centre of someone's universe. Someone who will always need you, who will always love you, who will always look up to you. It's called unconditional love.

You're not just a mum, you're you – and you are very important.

To Oscar,

You are the miracle of life.

If I could turn back the clocks to the moment I found out about you, I would tell my young, scared self to calm down, breathe and love every minute of what my body was doing to create you. I would tell myself not to care what people thought of me, to smile back at their curious looks as they walked by. I would run around telling the whole world about you and I'd walk with confidence into the book store and pick this book up. I'd tell myself to stop being anxious, to just be me and to trust my heart from the moment I heard your heartbeat.

Having you at nineteen made me who I am today, the mother I am to you, the wife that I now am to your father. To see life through your eyes has awoken my whole self to a greater appreciation of all humankind, all that we can achieve through love and kindness, and to accept that no one is perfect. Perfection and motherhood are two separate words that cannot sit together in the same sentence. You know that. But no matter how imperfect I am, I will love and need you, as you do me. Every mistake and challenge we go through in life, we will go through together. There will be no difference to my love for you than if you'd come eleven years later, when I was ready. All I wish is that I had put more energy into finding joy more quickly, and spending less time worrying about whether I was able, capable, brave enough to mother you.

Growing up pregnant with you was a journey that I would go through again, because it taught me so much more than a university course, than staying out partying, than turning night into day. You are the greatest teacher I could ever have hoped for, and it is wonderful to be growing up with you by my side for the rest of our lives. You created a revolution in my life, in your dad's life. We try so much harder because of you. You saved me from the person I was becoming, but I found my full self because of you. You are the beauty of life. You are my tiny miracle.

Believe in love

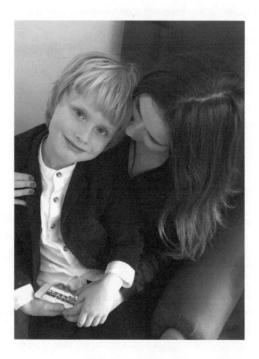

Resources

Here are some recommended sites that can support you:

tommys.org/pregnancy – Tommy's can support you with information on your pregnancy journey, answering questions with their symptom checker and reading case studies of other people's pregnancy journeys.

bestbeginnings.org.uk – Gives parents of all backgrounds the knowledge and confidence they need to look after their own mental and physical health whilst offering support on how to give your child the best start. Their 'Baby Buddy' app guides you through your pregnancy and the first six months of your baby's life.

girlsoutloud.org.uk – A resource and support network for young mums to join various programmes to regain confidence, self-belief, emotional resilience and a positive self image.

brook.org.uk – Run by confidential sexual health and wellbeing experts, this is a free resource to support you and answer any questions you may have.

familylives.org.uk – A national family support charity providing help and support in all aspects of family life.

littlelullaby.org.uk – Advice for young parents and a place where you can speak to other like minded young mums.

tpsp.ie – The Teen Parents Support Programme is a supportive site for young mums in Ireland who tailor their programme to your individual needs.

ypsn.ca – Young Parents Support Network in Canada is there to support and empower young parent families.

youngpregnantandparenting.org.au – Made up of health care providers, educators, social workers and community members from across Australia. They support pregnant and parenting young people to make the right choices and create the best outcomes for themselves and their children.

youngmomsupport.co.za – Young Mom Support in South Aftrica aiming to provide a safe, healthy and non-judgmental environment for young mothers of all races, cultures, religions and family situations to socialise with their children.

plannedparenthood.org – US-based health care provider Planned Parenthood delivers vital reproductive health care, sex education and information to millions of people worldwide. It is also available in Spanish.

generationher.org – Based in California this company helps to empower young mums and their children by connecting them to a supportive community of like-minded mothers. It also offers mentoring to equip you with the desired life skills that will ultimately impact your future in a positive way.

Acknowledgements

Thank you to Martin Wagner and Maria Pinter for their enthusiasm, guidance and insight and to all at Pinter & Martin for supporting me to complete the book I longed to write. You have made writing this book a joy.

Emma Grundy-Haigh, my editor – thank you for your patience and insightful editorial notes on my drafts, they have been invaluable.

Thank you midwife Anna Byrom, for your professional input and guidance, helping me to complete this book and provide valuable support for pregnant women out there.

Gary, my husband. Thank you for your loving encouragement and the support you have given me to accomplish this. I am forever grateful.

Thank you to my dysfunctional family whose issues feed my imagination. I love you all.

The Curleys – thank you for the loving support you have shown to me.

The McMasters – thank you for being there for me.

Thank you to my Mum, Rachael McLean, Carol Dunne and Sadie Dunne for their encouragement, for reading my manuscript and offering suggestions.

Cyclebox Squad – you continue to lift me and surround me with tools to lead a fuller, healthier life giving me energy to complete this book.

To everyone out there who has loved Oscar in their own way.

Thank YOU so much for buying this book. I truly appreciate it and hope you have enjoyed it.